**Opht
Note**

Ophthalmology Notes

Robert G. Small, M.D.

Professor of Ophthalmology
Dean A. McGee Eye Institute
The University of Oklahoma
Oklahoma Health Sciences Center
Oklahoma City, Oklahoma

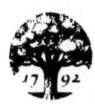

J.B. Lippincott Company Philadelphia
London   Mexico City   New York
St. Louis   São Paulo   Sydney

Acquisitions Editor: William Burgower
Developmental Editor: Delois Patterson
Manuscript Editor: Patrick O'Kane
Art Director: Tracy Baldwin
Design Coordinator: Don Shenkle
Designer: William Boehm
Production Supervisor: J. Corey Gray
Production Coordinator: Charlene Catlett Squibb
Compositor: General Graphic Services
Printer/Binder: R.R. Donnelley & Sons Company

Copyright © 1986, by J. B. Lippincott Company. All rights reserved. No part of this book may be used or reproduced in any manner whatsoever without written permission except for brief quotations embodied in critical articles and reviews. Printed in the United States of America. For information write J. B. Lippincott Company, East Washington Square, Philadelphia, Pennsylvania 19105.

6 5 4 3 2 1

Library of Congress Cataloging-in-Publication Data
Small, Robert G.
 Ophthalmology notes.

 Bibliography: p.
 Includes index.
 1. Ophthalmology.   I. Title.   [DNLM: 1. Eye Diseases. WW100 S635o]
 RE45.S63   1986   617.7   86-83
 ISBN 0-397-50738-0

The author and publisher have exerted every effort to ensure that drug selection and dosage set forth in this text are in accord with current recommendations and practice at the time of publication. However, in view of ongoing research, changes in government regulations, and the constant flow of information relating to drug therapy and drug reactions, the reader is urged to check the package insert for each drug for any change in indications and dosage and for added warnings and precautions. This is particularly important when the recommended agent is a new or infrequently employed drug.

To Claudia and Dia

Foreword

Dr. Robert Small has provided us a neatly packaged synopsis of clinical ophthalmology that succinctly and clearly provides a source of "core information" for physicians, students, and paramedical personnel. He has carefully outlined this information in a narrative style that is easily read and comprehended by those who are not familiar with the usual ophthalmologic jargon.

Thomas E. Acers, M.D.

Preface

Ophthalmology Notes is for you: the clinician, student, or medical professional.

Part 1 shows you how to examine and treat patients with acute conditions of the eye. About 5% of all who seek emergency care do so because of ocular symptoms.

Part 2 has a chapter for each major division of ophthalmology. These chapters, begun as lecture notes and revised over 20 years of teaching, make it easy for you to gain a working knowledge of ophthalmology. It is best to learn a few facts well. Thus, this handbook is shorter than most texts. Major topics are described briefly but in enough depth to give you a good foundation in diseases of the eye. Other conditions are defined in the glossary. *Italics* indicate that you can find a discussion of the entity by consulting the index.

Some common misunderstandings about the eye are noted in Chapter 18.

Memory experts say we learn best by forming mental images. The illustrations are designed to help you form those images.

There is an extensive literature in ophthalmology. The bibliography suggests some of the most important sources of additional information.

Whatever your work is in ophthalmology, may it be rewarding to you and of benefit to those who need eye care!

Robert G. Small, M.D.

Acknowledgments

I am indebted to the following reviewers of the text: Thomas E. Acers, M.D.; Hal D. Balyeat, M.D.; Tullos O. Coston, M.D.; James C. Hays, M.D.; Ronald M. Kingsley, M.D.; Wayne F. March, M.D.; Robert E. Nordquist, Ph.D.; James M. Richard, M.D.; J. James Rowsey, M.D.; Robert P. Shaver, M.D.; Gene R. Smith, Jr., M.D, and C. P. Wilkinson, M.D.

Morton F. Goldberg, M.D., made valuable suggestions in the preparation of the manuscript.

Stan Jacobson, assisted by Shelly Moody and Nancy Ryan, did the illustrations and lettering.

Special thanks to Ann C. Hyde, who helped me revise and correct the manuscript innumerable times.

My appreciation to the following at the J. B. Lippincott Company: Robert W. Reinhardt, Delois Patterson, Tracy Baldwin, and Patrick O'Kane.

Contents

PART 1   **Examination; Emergencies; Pharmacology**

1. Examination of the Eye *3*
2. Diagnosis and Treatment of Eye Emergencies *17*
3. Ocular Pharmacology and Therapeutics *34*

PART 2   **Basic Ophthalmology**

4. External Disease: Conjunctiva, Cornea, and Sclera *43*
5. Uveitis (Iritis, Iridocyclitis, Choroiditis) *51*
6. Glaucoma *55*
7. Vascular Diseases of the Eye *60*
8. Optics and Refraction *70*
9. Strabismus *78*
10. Cataract *85*
11. Neuro-Ophthalmology *89*
12. Eyelid, Lacrimal, and Orbital Diseases and Surgery *103*
13. The Cornea *115*
14. The Retina and Vitreous *120*
15. The Eye in Systemic Disease *129*
16. Special Diagnostic Studies *134*
17. Lasers in Ophthalmology *138*
18. Common Misunderstandings About the Eye *140*

Glossary *143*
Annotated Bibliography *169*
Index *171*

Part 1 Examination; Emergencies; Pharmacology

1 Examination of the Eye

History

Ask the patient about the presenting eye complaint: onset, duration, extent of visual loss, pain, redness, discharge, and so on. Then inquire about previous loss of vision in either eye or previous eye injury, disease, infection, or surgery. Was there, for example, a "lazy eye" (*strabismus*) in childhood? Is there a family history of eye disease? Which is the better eye? Was the present loss of vision sudden (suggests vascular disease) or gradual (suggests *cataract* or *macular degeneration*)? Is systemic disease present that could affect the eyes? Has poor vision affected normal activity? Is vision adequate for driving a car? (Requirements vary, but 20/40 is a common minimum visual requirement.) Is the patient **legally blind?** (20/200 or less in the better eye or a visual field of 20° or less in the better eye)? Patients are pleased to learn that income tax reduction, travel discounts, talking books, and other benefits are available to the legally blind.

Symptoms

Red eye—Frequent causes are *conjunctivitis, subconjunctival hemorrhage, keratitis, uveitis, glaucoma, injuries,* and *foreign bodies.*
Visual loss with pain—*Injuries, keratitis, uveitis,* and *acute glaucoma* are common causes of visual loss with pain.
Painless visual loss—Some causes are *retinal vein or retinal artery occlusion, vitreous hemorrhage,* and *retinal detachment.* (See also Chapter 2, page 33.)

3

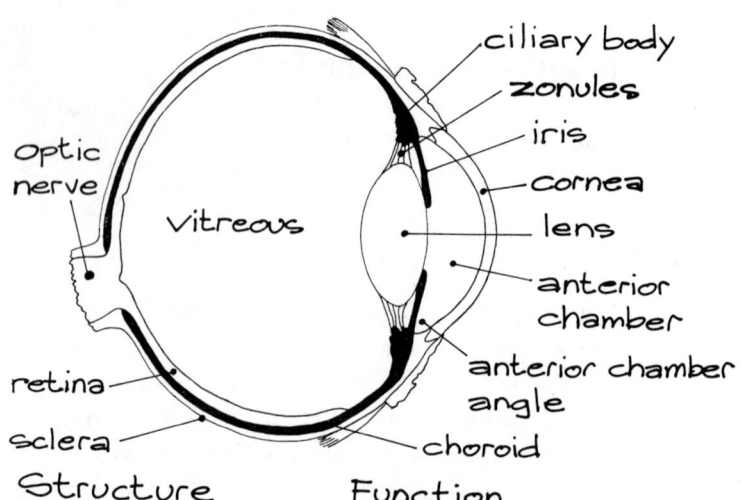

Structure Function

Cornea - Protects ocular structures; refracts light; permeable to topical eye medication.

Anterior chamber - Contains aqueous which transmits and refracts light, nourishes lens, and drains into anterior chamber angle.

Iris - Regulates amount of light entering eye.

Lens - Refracts light; changes shape during accommodation.

Zonules - Support lens; loosen lens capsule during accommodation.

Ciliary body - Secretes aqueous; contracts during accommodation.

Choroid - Supplies blood to outer retina.

Vitreous - Maintains shape of eye; transmits light.

Retina - Photoreceptors change light to nerve impulses; axons of ganglion cell layer make up optic nerve.

Optic nerve - Transmits visual impulse.

Sclera - Protective wall of eye.

Examination of the Eye

Double vision—Diplopia in a patient with no history of strabismus is a serious symptom that suggests intracranial involvement of the third, fourth, or sixth cranial nerve. It is discussed under *extraocular muscle palsy* in Chapter 9. Double vision also occurs in *Graves' disease* and *blowout fractures of the orbit*. Double vision in just one eye (**monocular diplopia**) can result from optical defects in the cornea or lens. The patient may report three images: one from the sound eye and two from the affected eye.

Proptosis—Bulging of one or both eyes occurs with or without swelling of the eyelids. Causes are *Graves' disease, orbital tumors, orbital pseudotumors, orbital cellulitis, cavernous sinus thrombosis, carotid-cavernous fistula,* and *mucormycosis*. Proptosis and orbital diseases are discussed in Chapter 12.

Pain in a "quiet" eye—If the eye is not red and vision is normal, some causes of eye pain are *migraine,* tension or vascular headache, *Horton syndrome, asthenopia,* and sinusitis.

Foreign body sensation—Evert the upper and lower eyelids and look for a *conjunctival foreign body*. Other causes are *corneal foreign body, corneal abrasion, keratitis, conjunctivitis,* and *dry eyes* from reduced tear secretion.

Photophobia—Any eye inflammation may be associated with sensitivity to light. Other causes are albinism, opacities in the ocular media, trigeminal neuropathy, and various neurologic conditions.

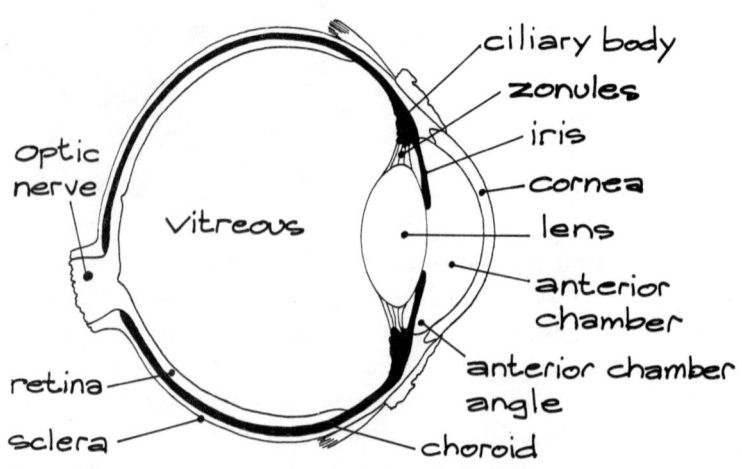

Structure	Abnormalities

<u>Cornea</u> - Keratitis; abrasion; ulcer; perforation.

<u>Anterior chamber</u> - Inflammation; hypopion; hemorrhage; hyphema; blocked angle leads to acute glaucoma.

<u>Iris</u> - Iritis; rubeosis iridis.

<u>Lens</u> - Cataract; dislocation.

<u>Zonules</u> - Weakening from injury or disease leads to dislocation of lens.

<u>Ciliary body</u> - Cyclitis; hyposecretion leads to hypotony.

<u>Choroid</u> — Choroiditis; degeneration; melanoma.

<u>Vitreous</u> — Hemorrhage; infection; traction leads to retinal detachment.

<u>Retina</u> — Degeneration; hemorrhage; detachment; abnormal new vessels; retinoblastoma.

<u>Optic nerve</u> - Optic neuritis; optic atrophy; glioma.

<u>Sclera</u> - Scleritis; ectasia.

Tearing—Tearing is caused by any eye infection, irritation or pain in the distribution of the fifth cranial nerve. Chronic *unilateral tearing* with discharge suggests mechanical obstruction of the nasolacrimal drainage system.

Red-rimmed crusted eyes—Chronic *blepharitis* is caused by *Staphylococcus* infection or seborrhea; it is also caused by allergy, *Demodex folliculorum*, malnutrition, rosacea, and poor hygiene.

Haloes—Haloes classically occur in *narrow-angle glaucoma* due to edema of the cornea. More often they are physiologic or the result of various optical effects, such as corneal edema or *cataract*.

Night blindness—Patients often complain that they have trouble seeing in the dark, but this rarely indicates eye disease. Retinal degeneration in *retinitis pigmentosa* produces profound night blindness. Obtain an *electroretinogram (ERG)* if symptoms are severe.

Metamorphopsia—Distortion of the shape of objects suggests *central serous chorioretinopathy* or other macular disturbance.

Photopsia—Seeing flashes of light is usually a harmless effect of vitreous traction on the retina. Occasionally the cause is *migraine*, early retinal detachment, or an occipital lesion.

Spots before the eyes—Vitreous floaters are usually normal. The sudden appearance of a cloud of floaters may indicate a *retinal detachment, retinal hole, vitreous detachment,* or *vitreous hemorrhage.*

Examination; Emergencies; Pharmacology

Twitching of the eyelids (myokymia)—This is common in people who are tired or under stress, or who have a high caffeine intake.

Visual Acuity

Visual acuity is the essential index of ocular function. Begin every eye examination by determining the central and peripheral vision in each eye.

Central Vision

The corresponding letters on each line of the Snellen chart (20/30, 20/40, 20/200, etc.) produce the same retinal image if viewed at the distance indicated by the denominator. To see Alcor, the tiny star just above the second star in the handle of the Big Dipper, you must have the same visual acuity as is needed

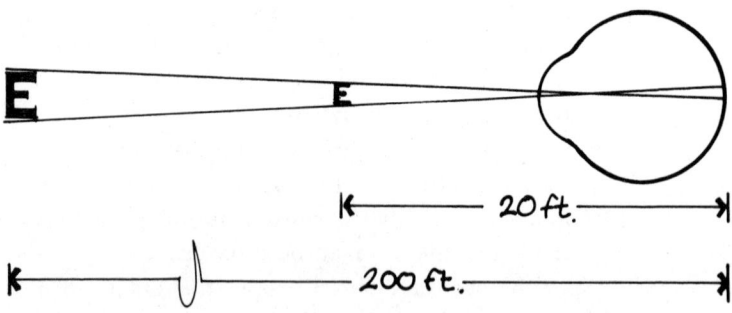

The normal eye can see the 20/200 E at 200 feet and the 20/20 E at 20 feet.

Examination of the Eye

to recognize the 20/20 E at 20 feet and the 20/200 E at 200 feet. This is 20/20 vision.

The Snellen notation 20/40 means that at 20 feet from the chart the patient can only read the 20/40 line, which a person with normal vision can read at 40 feet. The numerator gives the distance in feet between the patient and the chart. The denominator gives the distance at which a person with normal vision can see the line in question. Converted to metric notation, 20/20 is 6/6, 20/40 is 6/12 and 20/200 is 6/60.

If the patient cannot read the large 20/200 E, hold up your fingers and record the distance at which the patient can count them. This is **finger count vision**. With less vision, record the patient's ability to see your hand move (**hand motion vision**), to determine the direction of projected light (**light projection**), or to merely perceive light (**light perception**). If there is total blindness, use the term **no light perception** (**NLP**). Note if the eye has been enucleated.

A chart with no record of visual acuity may lead to medicolegal problems. Record the best possible visual acuity—with glasses, if they help. See if a pinhole disc in front of the eye sharpens vision. A pinhole disc improves vision almost as much as glasses. If you do not check visual acuity, note the reason. For example, in the case of a penetrating injury, forceful opening of the eyelids might cause expulsion of the contents of the eye.

Often, a drop of local anesthetic will enable the patient to open the eyes. At the bedside use a reading

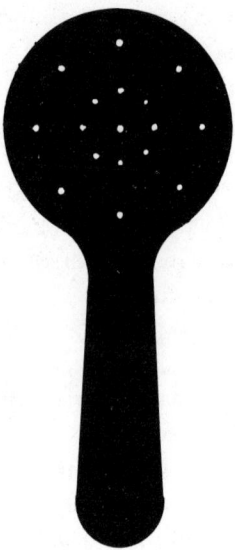

Pinhole disc

card. The ability to read newsprint at 14 inches indicates 20/40 vision.

Visual Field (Peripheral Vision)

To test peripheral vision have the patient look straight at you and count one or two fingers of your hand in each quadrant of the visual field (**confrontation field**). First test both eyes. Then test each eye separately with the other eye covered. In this way, unilateral or bilateral field defects are discovered without special equipment.

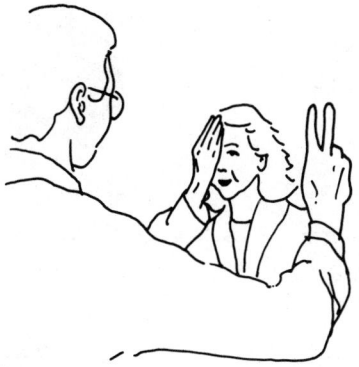

Confrontation visual field examination

Visual Field Defects

Field defects in one eye suggest lesions of the retina or optic nerve on that side. Central field defects suggest *optic neuritis* or macular disease. The patient sees an empty space where the letters on the Snellen chart should be. An early *retinal detachment* produces a partial loss of the upper or lower visual field in one eye. *Branch occlusion of a retinal artery or retinal vein* produces a field defect in one eye corresponding to the area of ischemic retina. *Chronic simple glaucoma* produces insidious contraction of the visual field. An **altitudinal field defect** is loss of the upper or lower half of the visual field.

Field defects in both eyes reflect damage to the optic chiasm, optic tract, lateral geniculate body, op-

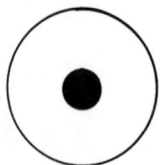

Central scotoma as in optic neuritis or macular degeneration.

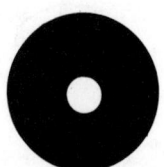

Peripheral constriction as in advanced glaucoma, retinitis pigmentosa, or hysteria.

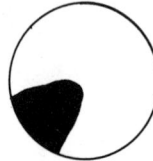

Segmental defect as in branch retinal vein or artery occlusion.

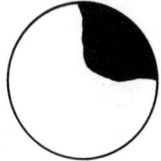

Quadrantic defect as in early retinal detachment.

Examples of monocular visual field defects

tic radiation, or occipital cortex. When charted, these **homonymous hemianopic or quadrantic defects** look like half or quarter pieces of pie symmetrically located in the right or left half of each visual field.

Examination of the External Eye

Use a penlight and loupe to examine the external eye. It is customary to examine the right eye first. Inspect the eyelids, eyelashes, conjunctiva, cornea, anterior chamber, iris, pupil, lacrimal system, and

Examination of the Eye

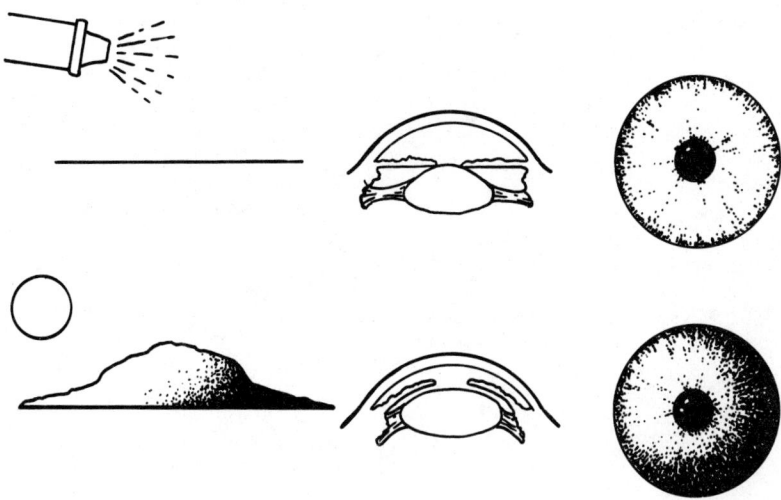

A penlight in the plane of the iris should result in uniform illumination. When the chamber is shallow the iris opposite the light is in shadow.

so on. Study eye movements and pupil reactions. See if the anterior chamber looks shallow. Evert the upper and lower eyelids and inspect the palpebral conjunctiva.

Ophthalmoscopic Examination

Dilate the pupils with 1% tropicamide if they are too small for ophthalmoscopy. Use caution in dilating the pupils in the following circumstances:

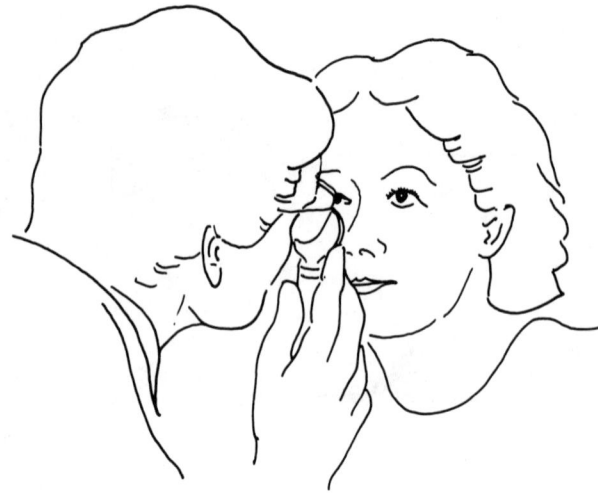

Direct ophthalmoscopy

1. The anterior chamber is shallow, suggesting undiagnosed *narrow-angle glaucoma*.
2. Neurologic disease or injury is present.
3. The patient has an iris-supported *intraocular lens*.
4. The eye is severely injured.

Observe the red pupil reflex through the +5 lens of the ophthalmoscope about 6 inches from the dilated pupil. This reveals *cataracts* and *vitreous floaters*. Then refocus and study the optic disc, retinal vessels, macula and retina. The **ocular media** are the transparent structures through which light passes to reach the retina. If you cannot see the retina, try to determine which structure is clouded. The opacity may be in the cornea, anterior chamber, lens, or vitreous.

The miotic pupil of the infant must be dilated for ophthalmoscopic examination. Children usually have large pupils with crystal-clear media. The retinal arterioles in youth are often tortuous. With age they narrow and become straight. In all ages the retinal arterioles are slightly smaller in diameter than the retinal venules.

Pulsation of retinal veins is not abnormal, since intraocular pressure is close to pressure in the ven-

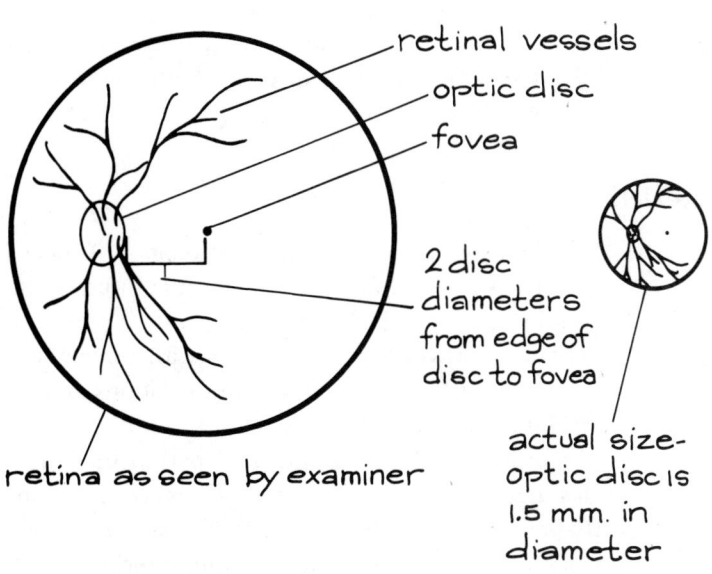

Retinal landmarks

ules. Retinal arteriolar pulsation, except in children, is usually pathologic, as in glaucoma, when intraocular pressure is abnormally high, or in carotid occlusive disease, when retinal arterial pressure is abnormally low.

The pupil gets smaller with age and the ocular media become cloudy due to changes in the lens and vitreous. Patients often describe annoying strands or cobwebs, which are usually normal *vitreous floaters*.

Study the optic disc for edema, cupping, pallor, and vascular abnormalities. Ophthalmoscopy often reveals the changes of *macular degeneration*, a common cause of visual loss in old age (Chapter 14). The ophthalmoscope is also valuable in detecting the vascular changes of hypertension, arteriosclerosis, diabetes (Chapter 7), and diseases of the retina and choroid (Chapter 14).

Abbreviations

Abbreviations abound in ophthalmology. VA means visual acuity. The following subscripts indicate the condition under which the acuity is tested: cc = with glasses; sc = without glasses; cl = with contact lenses; ph = with pinhole. Other abbreviations are *OD* = right eye, *OS* = left eye; *OU* = both eyes; *IOP* = intraocular pressure; *EOM* = extraocular muscles; *ET* = *esotropia;* *XT* = *exotropia*. Since each ophthalmology service has its own abbreviations and acronyms, care must be taken in communication with other physicians to avoid misunderstandings.

2 Diagnosis and Treatment of Eye Emergencies

Go through the following five steps to make a tentative diagnosis in all acute eye conditions:

1. **Take a history** of the presenting complaint and note any previous eye injury, eye disease, ocular surgery, or poor vision.
2. **Test the central and peripheral vision.**
3. **Examine the external eye and ocular adnexa** with a penlight and loupe. Then study the intraocular structures with an ophthalmoscope. Dilate the pupils if necessary, except as noted in Chapter 1.
4. **Stain the cornea with fluorescein** to reveal damage to the corneal epithelium (see p 23).
5. **Test the intraocular pressure** with the Schiøtz tonometer unless fluorescein reveals corneal damage. See Chapter 6 for a description of how to use the Schiøtz tonometer.

If the eye is irritated, instill a topical anesthetic. This affords temporary relief of pain and permits a better examination. Refer patients with recent loss of vision. Industrial accidents require referral, since an ophthalmologist's report is necessary for insurance benefits. Provide for follow-up care in writing so you will be sure your diagnosis is correct and your treatment effective.

Examination; Emergencies; Pharmacology

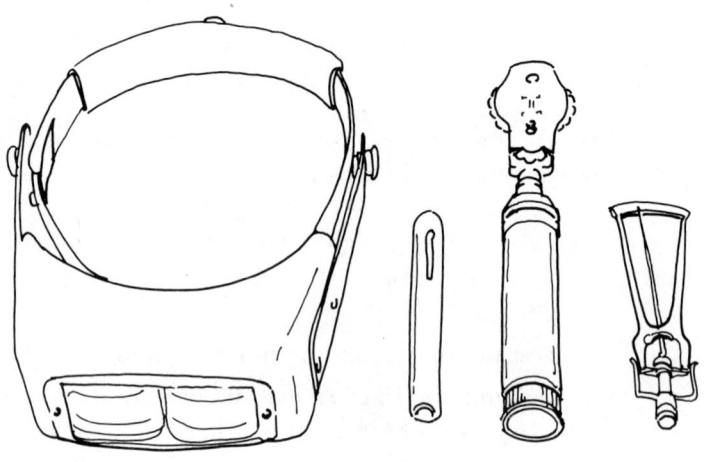

Basic equipment for eye examination: loupe; penlight; ophthalmoscope; tonometer

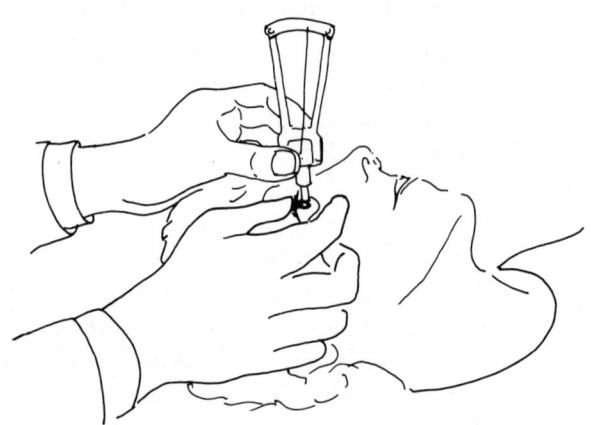

Schiotz tonometry

Diagnosis and Treatment of Eye Emergencies

How to Evaluate a Red Eye

The six conditions listed below account for almost all red eyes you will see. The five-step examination suggested above differentiates these entities.

Vision Normal

Acute conjunctivitis—The bulbar and palpebral conjunctiva are red, but the cornea remains clear.

Subconjunctival hemorrhage—There is sudden onset of painless, red discoloration of the bulbar conjunctiva.

Vision Usually Reduced

Eye injury—The history and external examination suggest the diagnosis.

Corneal disease or injury—Fluorescein stains the damaged corneal epithelium.

Acute glaucoma—The intraocular pressure is sharply elevated. The pupil is mid position or dilated. The cornea is cloudy.

Iritis—The aqueous is cloudy; the pupil is small or irregular.

Conjunctivitis

In conjunctivitis the eye is red, symptoms are mild, there is moderate discharge, and little or no loss of

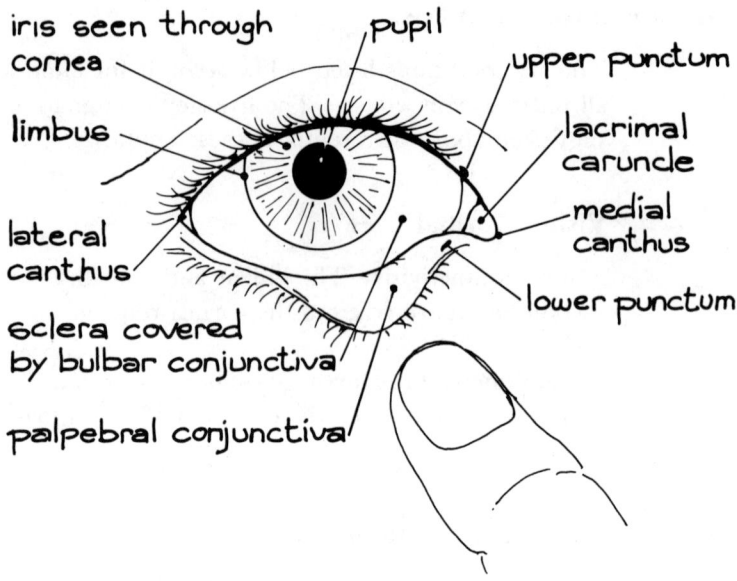

External eye - landmarks

vision. Treat with frequent instillation of sodium sulfacetamide or gentamicin eye drops. If symptoms persist after several days, refer. Profuse discharge suggests gonorrhea. Use caution, since conjunctivitis is often contagious. (See also Chapter 4.)

Subconjunctival Hemorrhage

The white conjunctiva is suddenly, painlessly stained with blood when a small conjunctival vessel ruptures. Part or all of the "white" of the eye is bright red, but this clears in 1 to 3 weeks without treatment. Subconjunctival hemorrhage is common in older people, but can occur at any age. It may follow vomiting, coughing, straining, or trauma but is often spontaneous.

Contusion of the Eye

Trauma from a rock, stick, or other object can cause a variety of ocular injuries. Corneal abrasion is common. Blood may cloud the aqueous or settle in the lower anterior chamber (*hyphema*). In an "eightball hemorrhage" the anterior chamber is filled with blood and the iris is obscured. All hyphemas should be under the immediate care of an ophthalmologist. Blunt trauma can cause retinal edema or detachment, choroidal tears, vitreous hemorrhage, damage to the macula or optic nerve, and late glaucoma. The same injury may produce an *orbital fracture* or rupture of the globe. Refer all patients who report loss of vision.

Orbital Fractures

Any blow near the eye can fracture the bony orbit. The injury varies in severity from massive disruption of the orbit to a crack in the orbital rim.

A **tripod fracture** has breaks at three sites in the orbital rim. Surgery is usually necessary.

In a **blowout fracture** the orbital floor is involved but the rim of the orbit is intact. Typically, the patient cannot elevate the eye on the injured side. A characteristic feature is numbness of the cheek or mouth from injury to the maxillary nerve. Swollen eyelids may hide the fracture. When the swelling subsides the patient will note double vision if ocular muscles are trapped in the fracture. The physician will be criticized if the diagnosis is missed on initial examination. If there is any possibility of fracture, get a Waters' view X-ray. Opacification of the maxillary antrum on the side of the injury suggests a blowout fracture. Laminograms or a CT scan may be necessary to show the fracture. Surgery is usually necessary if ocular muscles are trapped in the fracture but is often delayed until the swelling subsides. Carefully evaluate the eye, since ocular injury often accompanies orbital fractures.

Penetrating Injuries of the Eye

A great variety of objects can penetrate the cornea or sclera. The injury varies in severity from an inconspicuous wound to rupture of the eye. All penetrating injuries are serious because of the possibility of permanent loss of vision from infection, hemorrhage, or damage to the eye. A common appearance is a small purple mass of iris protruding from a corneal laceration with distortion of the pupil and a flat anterior chamber. Always get an X-ray to rule out a retained *intraocular foreign body*. Tell the X-ray technician not to position the patient face down, since doing so may increase eye damage. Emergency surgery is usually required, so put the patient on NPO. Penetrating wounds of the eye may extend into the cranium, so be alert for CNS symptoms and signs.

Laceration of the Eyelids

If a laceration crosses the eyelid margin or involves the tear duct system at the inner canthus of the eye, surgery by an ophthalmologist is required. Superficial lacerations may be closed at the discretion of the physician. If fat is seen bulging into the wound, the laceration has probably penetrated the orbit, with possible injury to deep adnexal structures. Rule out injury to the eye itself, which may not be immediately apparent. Lacerations of the upper eyelid may result in *blepharoptosis* if not properly repaired.

Corneal Disease and Injury

When the cornea is diseased or injured (Chapter 4), the patient usually complains of pain or the sensation of having a foreign body in the eye. Instill a drop of topical anesthetic. Moisten a *fluorescein strip* with saline and put a drop in the lower conjunctival fornix. Corneal abrasions and ulcers stain green. Superficial abrasions cause little or no loss of vision and heal in 1 or 2 days. Prescribe a topical antibiotic eye drop. Patch the eye. Give an oral analgesic for pain, but never prescribe local anesthetic eye drops. Refer if the lesion is large or does not heal in 1 or 2 days.

Look for the branching pattern pathognomonic

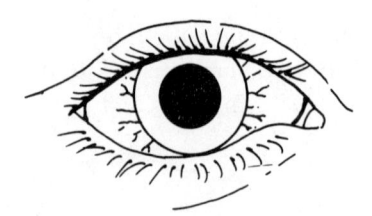

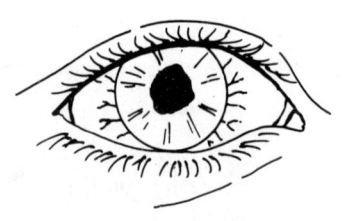

Acute glaucoma

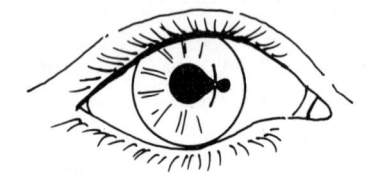

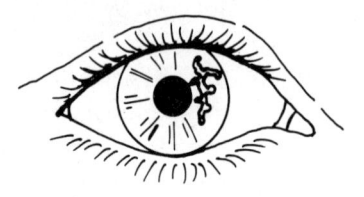

Acute iritis

Corneal laceration with iris prolapse

Herpetic keratitis

of *herpetic keratitis*. Refer these patients promptly, since herpetic keratitis can cause serious visual loss. Avoid eye drops that contain steroids if you suspect herpetic keratitis.

Foreign Bodies

Foreign bodies occur in the conjunctiva, cornea, or inside the eye.

Conjunctival foreign bodies are found anywhere on the bulbar or palpebral conjunctiva, but often under the upper eyelid with severe cor-

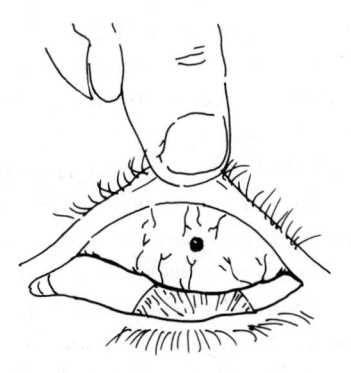

Foreign body under upper eyelid

neal irritation. Dramatic relief follows eversion of the upper eyelid and removal of the foreign body.

Corneal foreign bodies are often imbedded metal fragments from tools or machinery. After instilling a topical anesthetic, remove with a 20 gauge needle or spud using loupe magnification. Residual rust must be removed by an ophthalmologist with a motor-driven bur. Use caution if the center of the cornea is involved, since scarring here will blur vision.

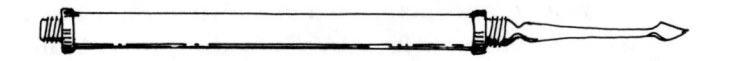

Foreign body spud

Intraocular foreign bodies can destroy the eye by secondary infection, by chemical damage—from iron (**siderosis**) or copper (**chalcosis**)—or by mechanical damage to ocular structures. Occasionally, small objects penetrate the eye at high speed, causing an inconspicuous wound and few immediate signs or symptoms. Serious problems usually occur soon, however. Get X-rays and consultation whenever there is any possibility of an intraocular foreign body. Blindness and litigation may follow if this diagnosis is missed.

Endophthalmitis

Bacteria or fungi introduced by penetrating wounds, during surgery, or following perforation of a *corneal ulcer* may cause septic inflammation of all the intraocular structures. The eye is red and painful, and the anterior chamber structures are obscured by pus. The patient must be hospitalized immediately for local and systemic antibiotic therapy and possible *vitrectomy*.

Ultraviolet Light Keratitis

Looking at a welder's torch or sunlamp can cause painful keratitis ("flashburn"). A drop or two of local anesthetic provides dramatic temporary relief, but do not prescribe these drops. Close inspection is necessary to see tiny dots in the cornea that stain with fluorescein (*superficial punctate keratitis*). The eyes are red and there is mild loss of vision. Treatment includes eyepatches, analgesics, sedatives for sleep, and antibiotic eye drops. Refer if symptoms do not improve in 24 hours.

Contact Lens Keratitis

Keratitis or corneal ulcer can be caused by overwearing of contact lenses, infection, poor hygiene, and warped, scratched, or ill-fitting *contact lenses* of any type. The patient complains of severe eye pain. Fluorescein stain reveals keratitis or ulcer. Topical anesthesia provides immediate relief, but do not prescribe these drops. Treatment is the same as for ultraviolet light keratitis. The contact lenses should be checked by the physician who prescribed them.

Chemical Burns of the Cornea

When an acid or alkali has come in contact with a patient's eyes, irrigate immediately and continuously with copious amounts of water. When possible instill a topical anesthetic and continue irrigating with normal saline until pH paper indicates neutralization. If the cornea remains clear, the prognosis is good. Persistent corneal clouding warrants hospitalization for continuous irrigation. Lye burns have a poor prognosis.

Iritis (Iridocyclitis; Uveitis)

The patient with iritis (Chapter 5) presents with redness of the eye at the limbus (*ciliary injection*), blurred vision, a small or irregular pupil, cloudy aqueous, and dull pain over the eyebrow. The view with an ophthalmoscope is hazy because the aqueous contains inflammatory cells and protein. Clumps of white cells may be seen on the back of the cornea, on the iris, or layered in the anterior chamber (*hypopyon*).

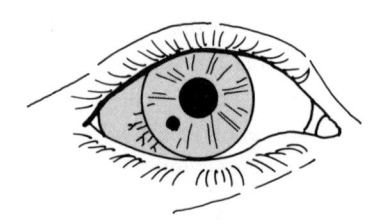

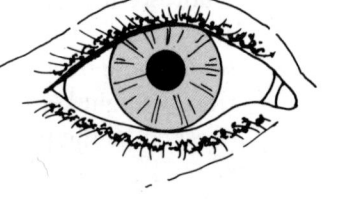

Corneal foreign body

Blepharitis

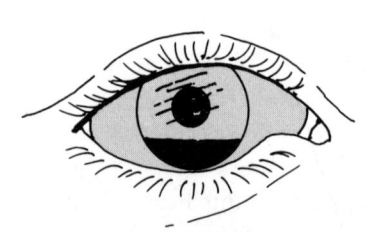

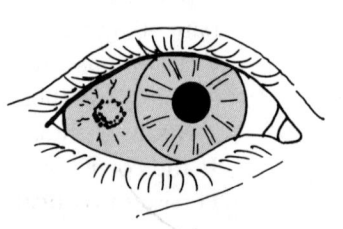

Contusion with corneal abrasion and hyphema

Episcleritis

Intraocular pressure is normal or moderately elevated. Refer when any kind of uveitis is suspected.

Scleritis

Scleritis and *episcleritis* appear as localized flat or raised areas of vascular engorgement over inflamed sclera. In episcleritis the pain is mild and the inflamed conjunctival vessels can be moved over the sclera by gentle finger pressure through the eyelid. In scleritis the pain is more severe and the inflamed vessels are immobile. Refer if scleritis is suspected (Chapter 4).

Acute Narrow-Angle Glaucoma

The patient with acute narrow-angle glaucoma (Chapter 6) typically has a red, painful, cloudy eye, loss of vision, and nausea and vomiting. Findings include sharply elevated intraocular pressure, a shallow anterior chamber, a cloudy cornea, and a fixed dilated or mid-dilated pupil. Inappropriate laparotomy may be done if abdominal pain, nausea and vomiting induced by the glaucomatous attack is misdiagnosed. Prompt laser *iridotomy* or surgical *iridectomy* is curative. Note that the more common *open-angle glaucoma* is painless and insidious in its onset.

Orbital Cellulitis

If the eyelids are swollen shut with infection and spreading cellulitis, hospitalize the patient and give

Orbital cellulitis

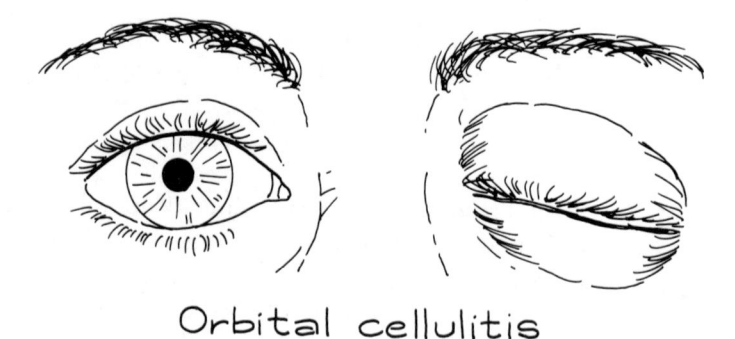

intensive intravenous antibiotics. Get X-rays and consultation, since surgical drainage or decompression of the orbit may be indicated. Orbital cellulitis is often secondary to acute sinusitis or dental infection, which when neglected may progress to meningitis or *cavernous sinus thrombosis*.

Mucormycosis

Mucor, a ubiquitous soil fungus, causes a fulminant, often fatal infection of the orbit, sinuses, nose, and brain in patients who have diabetic acidosis or immunodeficiency, or who are on cytotoxic or steroid medication. Pain, fever, *orbital cellulitis*, proptosis, purulent nasal discharge, and necrotic destruction of bone are characteristic. Prompt biopsy for diagnosis and *exenteration of the orbit* and sinuses may be lifesaving, since antifungal agents are usually not effective.

Acute dacryocystitis

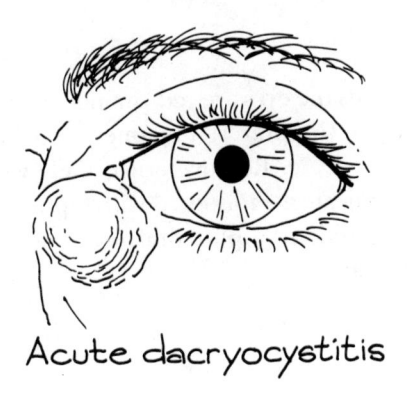

Acute Dacryocystitis

In acute dacryocystitis the infected lacrimal sac produces a red, tender mass on the side of the nose just below the inner canthus of the eye. The nasolacrimal duct is usually obstructed. Treat with warm compresses and antibiotics. Surgical drainage is often necessary.

Cavernous Sinus Thrombosis

Neglected facial, sinus, or dental infection, especially in diabetic, retarded, or debilitated individuals, may lead to cavernous sinus thrombophlebitis with *proptosis*, septicemia, coma, blindness, and death. Mortality is high even with intensive intravenous antibiotic therapy. Survivors may be blind. Predisposing conditions should be vigorously treated.

Blepharitis

In blepharitis the eyes are red-rimmed. Various causes are noted in Chapter 1. Treatment consists of eliminating the cause. Remove crusts daily with cotton-tipped applicators moistened with tap water and apply an antibiotic ophthalmic ointment such as sulfacetamide.

Stye (Hordeolum)

A stye is an abscess associated with an eyelash at the eyelid edge. It should be treated, like any abscess, with warm compresses and antibiotics. If it points, incise and drain. Chronic *blepharitis* is a predisposing condition.

Chalazion

A chalazion is a nodule in the tarsus that feels like a pea under the skin of the eyelid. It is due to obstruction of one of the tarsal (meibomian) glands. Secondary infection may occur. Surgery by an ophthalmologist is usually necessary.

Ophthalmia Neonatorum

The time of onset after birth gives a clue to the etiology of eye inflammation in the newborn. In the first 24 hours, mild conjunctivitis with scanty discharge is usually a reaction to prophylactic silver nitrate or antibiotic drops. A profuse purulent dis-

Chalazion

Stye

Acute conjunctivitis

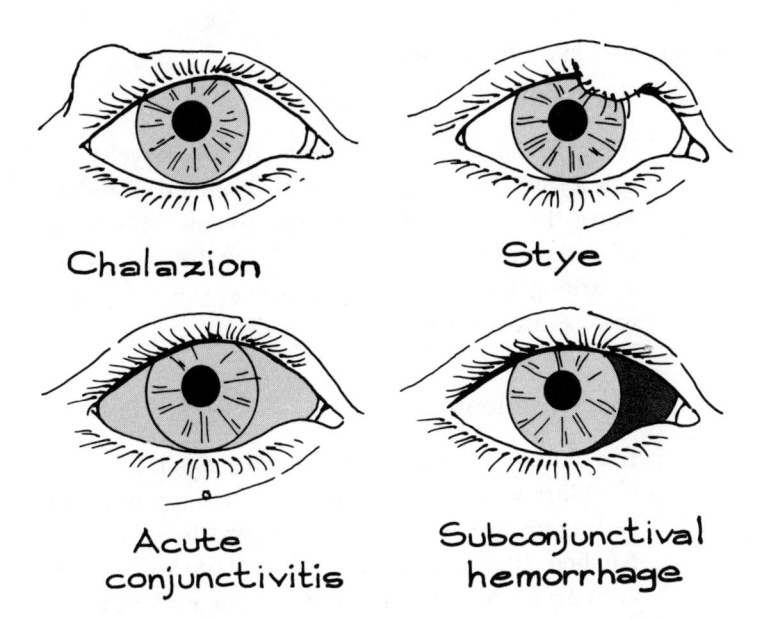

Subconjunctival hemorrhage

charge in the first few days of life suggests gonorrhea. Inflammation 5 to 7 days after birth is often a result of *chlamydial* infection (**inclusion conjunctivitis of the newborn**).

Painless Loss of Vision

Alarming painless loss of vision in a white "quiet" eye may be due to *central retinal vein occlusion, central retinal artery occlusion, retinal detachment, chorioretinitis, retinal or vitreous hemorrhage, optic neuritis,* the aura of *migraine,* intracranial or extracranial vascular occlusion, hysteria, or malingering. If the loss of vision is recent, refer to an ophthalmologist immediately since prompt treatment may preserve or improve vision.

3 Ocular Pharmacology and Therapeutics

Eye Drops and Eye Ointments

To Instill Eye Drops

Teach the patient to pull down the lower eyelid and put a drop or two in the lower conjunctival fornix. Have the patient close the eye for one minute so blinking and tearing will not wash out the drop. Avoid splashing the drop on the cornea, since doing so causes discomfort.

Eye Ointment

Eye ointment has more prolonged action than drops but blurs vision and is harder for patients to instill. Ointments are useful before bed or when the eye is patched. Instruct the patient to pull the lower eyelid away from the globe and instill about a quarter inch of ointment in the lower conjunctival fornix.

Caution

Patients sometimes have prescriptions refilled and use eye medication unsupervised for months or even years for themselves, family, and friends. Specify the duration of treatment and number of refills on your prescription.

Eye Patches

Patch both eyes and have the patient remain in a dark room for complete rest of an inflamed or injured eye. Patching just the affected eye is less effective, since movement of the pupil and muscles of the unpatched eye stimulates the pupil and muscles of the patched eye.

Compresses

Warm compresses are used for infection. Cold compresses are used for adnexal swelling after trauma or surgery. Eye patches soaked in warm or ice water are useful for compresses since they fit comfortably over the eyelids.

Cultures

Cultures are not routinely done in conjunctivitis, but are obtained in any eye-threatening infection, some corneal ulcers, and suspected fungal infection. Ideally, the physician obtains the specimen and transfers it immediately to a bacteriologic plate for incubation. Part of the specimen is placed on a glass slide and stained for microscopic study.

Antibiotic Eye Drops and Ointments

10% sulfacetamide is safe, usually not allergenic, relatively inexpensive, and a good first choice for the empiric treatment of conjunctivitis.

Gentamicin is an effective and widely used ophthalmic antibiotic.

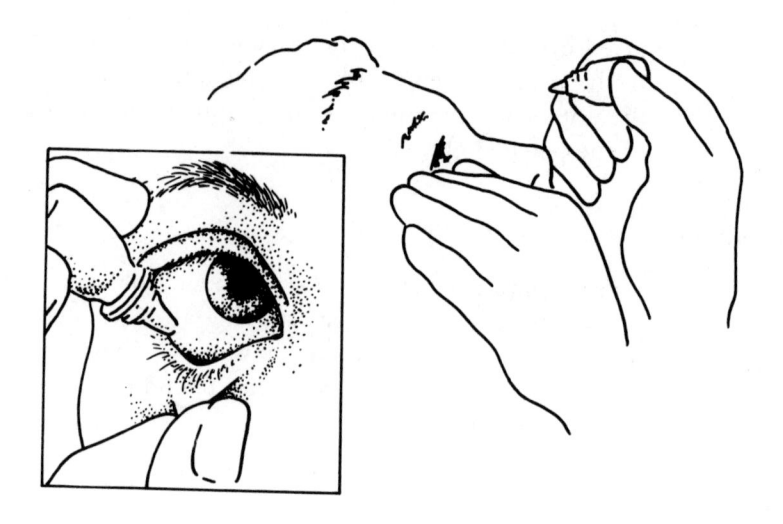

Administration of eye drops

Neomycin, polymyxin, and bacitracin are often found in combination. *Caution:* neomycin may be allergenic, especially with prolonged use.

Other commercially available ophthalmic antibiotics are gramacidin, sulfisoxazole, tetracycline, and tobramycin.

For the patient with conjunctivitis, prescribe antibiotic eye drops every hour while awake the first day, then every 2 to 3 hours while awake the next several days. If the patient shows no improvement, reevaluate or refer. Prolonged use of antibiotic eye drops may produce an irritative or chemical conjunctivitis. Systemic antibiotics are not necessary for most types of conjunctivitis.

Systemic Antibiotics

Oral or parenteral antibiotics are indicated for *gonorrheal ophthalmia,* endophthalmitis, *orbital cellulitis, dacryocystitis, cavernous sinus thrombosis,* and specific infections, such as *trachoma* and *tularemia.* It is usually not necessary to treat simple conjunctivitis with systemic antibiotics.

Subconjunctival and Intraocular Antibiotics

In severe infections, the ophthalmologist may inject antibiotics beneath the conjunctiva or into the eye itself.

Steroid Eye Drops and Ointments

Steroid eyedrops and ointments contain steroid alone or in combination with antibiotics. They are effective for temporary relief of allergic-bacterial conjunctivitis. Use with caution, however, since the use of steroid eye medication in herpetic and fungal keratitis may lead to corneal perforation. Long-term use of steroid eye medication can cause glaucoma and cataract.

Topical Anesthetic Eye Drops (Proparacaine, Tetracaine, Benoxinate)

Never prescribe topical anesthetic eye drops! Repeated use softens the corneal epithelium and interferes with corneal healing. Corneal scarring and loss of vision occur when these drops are used for days or weeks to ease the pain of corneal disease or injury.

Artificial Tears

Artificial tears contain polyvinyl alcohol or methylcellulose. These are usually safe for long-term use for dry eyes. Occasionally, preservatives in the drops irritate the eye. More than 20 varieties are available.

Eyewash (Collyrium)

Commercial eye-irrigating solutions are useful for the physician. Patients, however, do not need to rinse their eyes routinely. Boric acid solution, once thought to be good for the eyes, has no special value.

Decongestants

Frequent use of over-the-counter decongestants may irritate the eye. The active ingredient is tetrahydrozoline or phenylephrine. Occasional use is harmless. Zinc sulfate in some of these preparations is thought to have an astringent effect.

Cycloplegics

Cycloplegic eyedrops paralyze accommodation, for accurate *refraction* of the eye. They are also used to dilate the pupil for examination of the lens and retina. Dropper bottles containing cycloplegic medication have red tops.

Tropicamide 1% is the most commonly used cycloplegic. Instill one or two drops; repeat in 5 minutes. The pupil dilates in about 20 minutes. Near vision is blurred for several hours.
Cyclopentolate 1% is more potent and longer acting than tropicamide. The 2% solution has caused hallucinations in children.
Atropine 1% is the most potent cycloplegic. Its effects last for up to a week. Use only with the advice of an ophthalmologist.

Mydriatics

Mydriatics are eye medications that dilate the pupil, such as the cycloplegics above. A heavily pigmented iris requires a strong mydriatic or combination of mydriatics for dilation.

Phenylephrine hydrochloride 10% is a mydriatic with no cycloplegic effect. It is used to dilate the pupil for examination of the eye. *Caution:* hypertension and cardiac arrhythmias are possible side effects.

Glaucoma Medications

Timolol is often used first in open-angle glaucoma. It reduces aqueous secretion. The side effects associated with beta blockers, such as bradycardia and syncope, are occasionally seen. Timolol is contraindicated in asthmatics.

Dipivefrin is an epinephrine derivative that reduces aqueous secretion. It sometimes causes tachycardia and elevated blood pressure. Macular edema may occur in aphakic persons.

Pilocarpine improves aqueous outflow and for many years was the drug of choice for glaucoma. It constricts the pupil. By convention, it and other parasympathomimetic eye drops are dispensed in dropper bottles with green tops.

Methazolamide and **acetazolamide** are oral carbonic anhydrase inhibitors that reduce aqueous secretion.

Antiviral Eye Drops and Ointments

The following medications are used for herpes simplex keratitis: **trifluorothymidine, idoxuridine,** and **vidarabine.**

Part 2 Basic Ophthalmology

4 External Disease: Conjunctiva, Cornea, and Sclera

Conjunctivitis

The "white" of the eye becomes red in conjunctivitis because of superficial inflammation of the bulbar **conjunctiva** which covers the globe of the eye. You can demonstrate this superficial inflammation by moving the red bulbar conjunctiva by gentle finger pressure through the eyelid. In contrast, *uveitis* and *acute congestive glaucoma* are characterized by fixed, deep *ciliary injection*.

Mild conjunctivitis is sometimes called **acute catarrhal conjunctivitis**. Patients use the term "pink eye," and correctly assume it is contagious. Visual acuity remains good and the infection subsides in a few days with frequent administration of sulfacetamide or gentamicin eye drops.

Inflammation of the **palpebral conjunctiva**, which lines the inner surface of the eyelids, causes two common reactions. The first is **papillary conjunctivitis**, often caused by *Staphylococcus* and other pyogenic bacteria. Papillae are innumerable, 0.1-mm, vascularized tufts and have a characteristic velvety red appearance. Toxic substances, allergy, and continuous-wear soft contact lenses also produce papillary conjunctivitis. Itching suggests allergic conjunctivitis.

Follicular conjunctivitis, the second common palpebral conjunctival reaction, is characterized by innumerable translucent, 1-mm elevated nodules that give the appearance of a miniature cobblestone street. Follicles are lymphoid nodules produced by by viral, chlamydial, or granulomatous inflammation. The eye

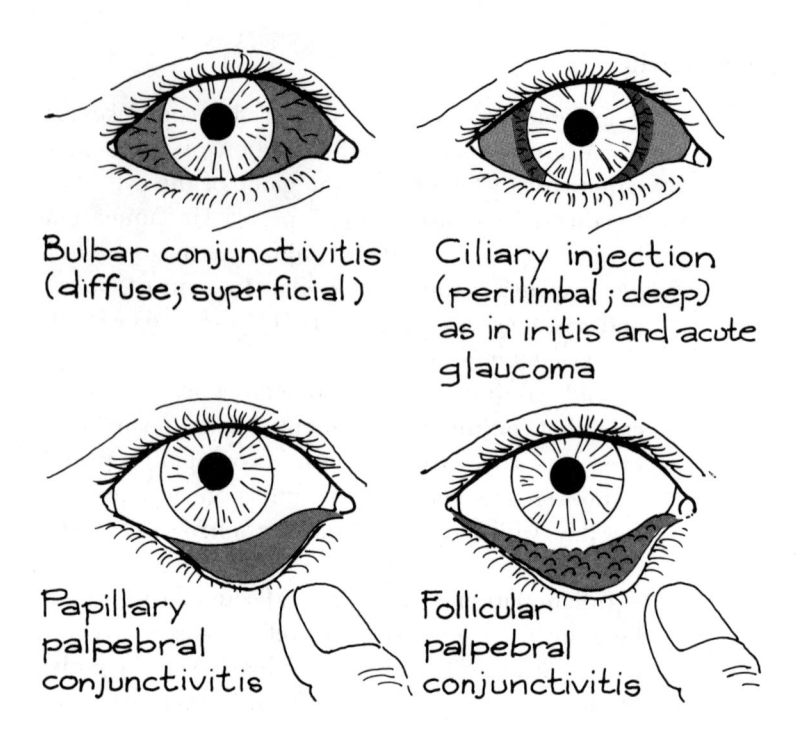

Bulbar conjunctivitis (diffuse; superficial)

Ciliary injection (perilimbal; deep) as in iritis and acute glaucoma

Papillary palpebral conjunctivitis

Follicular palpebral conjunctivitis

is red and the preauricular lymph nodes are often tender. Follicular conjunctivitis takes longer to subside than papillary conjunctivitis and is often associated with keratitis (**keratoconjunctivitis**).

Parinaud's oculoglandular syndrome historically meant *Leptothrix* infection. It now signifies conjunctivitis with visibly enlarged, tender preauricular lymph nodes, caused, in order of frequency, by cat scratch fever, tularemia, sporotrichosis, tuberculosis, syphilis, and coccidioidomycosis. Tularemia can be fatal, so conjunctivitis with visible preauricular nodes should be evaluated promptly.

Pharyngoconjunctival fever ("swimming pool conjunctivitis") is caused by adenoviruses type 3, 5, or 7. Children develop fever, sore throat, preauricular adenopathy, and conjunctivitis. These subside without specific treatment.

Epidemic keratoconjunctivitis (EKC) is highly contagious. It is caused by adenovirus type 8 or 19. Following conjunctivitis with pain, photophobia, and preauricular adenopathy, corneal infiltrates appear that may take months to clear. No antiviral agent will shorten this process.

Vernal conjunctivitis is a seasonal, recurrent, bilateral, allergic conjunctivitis of children that causes severe itching, giant cobblestone papillae of the tarsal conjunctiva, and pathognomonic white Trantas' dots at the corneal limbus. Treatment is with steroid

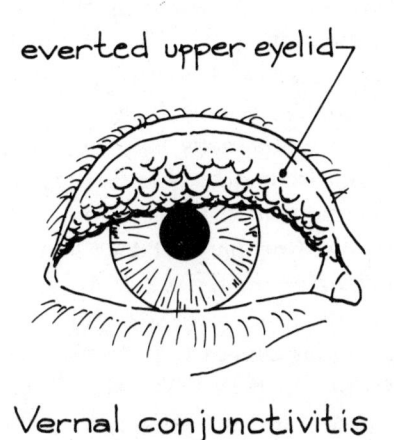

everted upper eyelid

Vernal conjunctivitis

and cromolyn eye drops. The disease may be recurrent for years but the prognosis is good.

Trachoma is a conjunctivitis of hot, dry climates caused by *Chlamydia trachomatis*. An estimated half billion people are affected, making it one of the most widespread diseases in the world and a leading preventable cause of blindness. Papillae and follicles of the upper tarsal conjunctiva lead to scarring, upper eyelid *entropion, trichiasis,* and scarring of the upper cornea (**pannus**). Topical and systemic tetracycline are effective but millions suffer loss of vision because of lack of treatment.

Inclusion conjunctivitis, also called swimming-pool conjunctivitis, is a chlamydial conjunctivitis related to trachoma, lymphogranuloma venereum, and psittacosis. It may be venereal in young adults and occurs in infants infected during birth.

Gonorrheal ophthalmia is characterized by a profuse yellow-green purulent conjunctival exudate. Get an anaerobic culture, examine a stained smear, and treat immediately with parenteral and topical penicillin. Be careful, since the disease is highly infectious.

Chronic conjunctivitis may be infectious, irritative, allergic, idiopathic, or associated with poor hygiene, poor nutrition, rosacea, or blepharitis. It is common in old people with dry eyes. Prolonged use of steroid or antibiotic eye drops may perpetuate conjunctivitis.

Membranous conjunctivitis is classically, but now rarely, caused by diphtheria. More commonly it results from any severe bacterial or viral infection or Stevens Johnson disease. If the membrane is peeled off, the conjunctiva will come with it, leaving a raw, bleeding surface.

Pseudomembranes may be removed without bleeding and occur in less severe forms of the conditions associated with membranous conjunctivitis.

Corneal Injury and Inflammation

(See also Chapter 13)

Corneal Ulcer

Stain the cornea with fluorescein to detect corneal disease or injury. Areas of loss of corneal epithelium stain bright green. Corneal ulcers may follow abrasions or contact lens wear. Debilitated or neglected patients are apt to develop a corneal ulcer following untreated infection by *Staphylococcus, Pseudomonas, Pneumococcus,* and other organisms.

The classic picture is of a serpiginous or central corneal ulcer with a **hypopyon**. A **hypopyon** is an accumulation of pus which may or may not be sterile layered in the bottom of the anterior chamber. The corneal ulcer may progress to perforation of the eye. Obtain corneal scrapings from the ulcer for a stained smear and culture. Treatment includes topical, subconjunctival, and systemic antibiotics, and a conjunctival flap operation if perforation of the cornea is threatened.

Superficial punctate keratitis (SPK) is characterized by multiple, tiny, corneal defects that are visible without fluorescein stain. These defects may be caused

Some acute corneal abnormalities

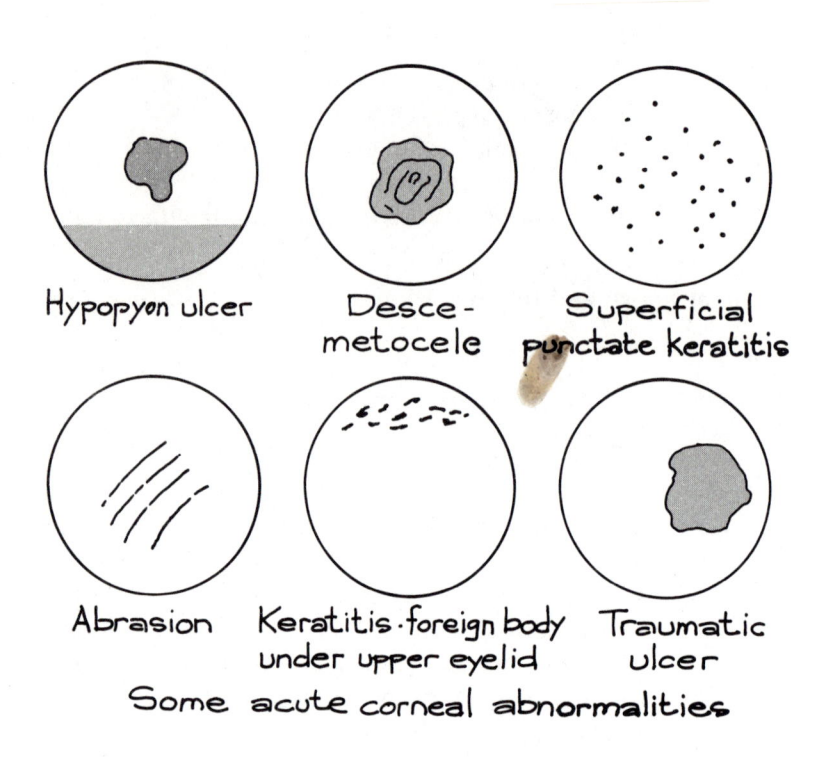

- Hypopyon ulcer
- Descemetocele
- Superficial punctate keratitis
- Abrasion
- Keratitis - foreign body under upper eyelid
- Traumatic ulcer

by certain adenoviruses or may represent a specific chronic keratitis described by Thygeson. More generally, SPK also means superficial corneal erosions that stain with fluorescein. These erosions can be caused by any corneal irritation, such as adenovirus infection, neomycin or other chemical toxicity, *contact lenses*, ultraviolet light, *blepharitis*, or *keratoconjunctivitis sicca*. Painful recurrent corneal erosions may be hereditary or may follow corneal abrasions.

Herpetic or dendritic keratitis is an important viral disease of the cornea caused by the herpes simplex virus (HSV). This ubiquitous virus (responsible for fever sores around the mouth) causes keratitis when host resistance decreases. Fluorescein stain reveals a pathognomonic branching or "dendritic" lesion following the distribution of corneal nerves. Permanent loss of vision may result. Treatment is debridement of the cornea by an ophthalmologist followed by trifluorthymidine eye drops. Steroid eye drops are contraindicated because they may result in corneal perforation. Herpetic keratitis in the newborn is an extreme emergency, since death from cerebral involvement is likely. Cesarean section is indicated in a mother with herpetic cervicitis.

Ophthalmic herpes zoster is a trigeminal ganglionitis caused by the varicella zoster virus (VZV). Painful inflammation follows the distribution of the ophthalmic nerve: eye, eyelids, forehead, nose, and upper face. Complications include damage to the skin and eyelids, *keratitis, uveitis,* alopecia, and postherpetic neuralgia.

Fungal corneal ulcers often follow injuries on the farm or in the garden. The fungus produces an indolent, destructive corneal ulcer. Steroid medication increases susceptibility to fungal keratitis. Treatment with topical pimaricin or amphotericin-B may be useful.

Diseases of the Sclera

Deep (nodular) scleritis is a painful scleral inflammation related to the collagen diseases. There is deep vascular engorgement over the affected areas of the

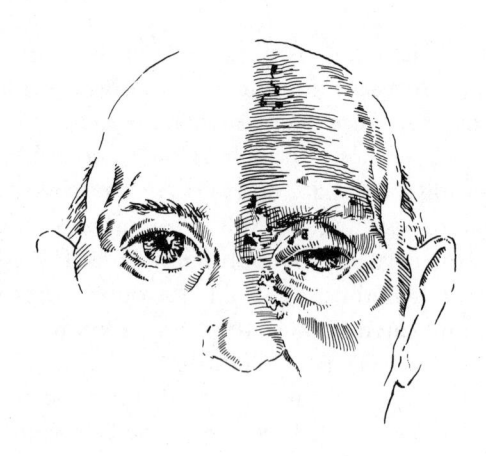

Herpes zoster ophthalmicus

sclera. Anterior chamber inflammation may be present. The eye may become blind in spite of systemic steroid therapy.

Scleromalacia perforans is a painless scleritis in which the blue ciliary body and choroid bulge through thinned sclera (**scleral ectasia**). This scleral necrosis is associated with rheumatoid arthritis and may destroy the eye.

Episcleritis is a superficial, mildly painful, scleral inflammation of uncertain etiology. The conjunctival vessels are red over the inflamed sclera. The disorder is self-limited and has a good prognosis.

5 Uveitis (Iritis, Iridocyclitis, Choroiditis)

The uvea comprises the middle vascular layer of the eye: iris, ciliary body, and choroid. Anterior uveitis is iritis or iridocyclitis. Posterior uveitis is choroiditis. The red eye of iritis is due to engorged vessels in the sclera close to the corneal limbus (**ciliary injection**) in contrast to the superficial redness of conjunctivitis.

Iritis

Iritis (**Anterior nongranulomatous uveitis; iridocyclitis**) is characterized by a red, painful eye with blurred vision. The etiology is usually unknown, although immunologic factors are thought to be important. Various microorganisms may also be responsible.

Inflamed vessels in the iris and ciliary body leak protein and inflammatory cells into the aqueous, making it cloudy. Close inspection with a slit of light reveals protein and cells in the aqueous. The effect is like a beam of sunlight shining through a chink in the roof of a dusty attic (**aqueous flare and cells**). Clumps of inflammatory cells on the corneal endothelium are called **keratic precipitates (k.p.)**; on the stroma of the iris, **Busacca nodules**; and on the pupillary margin of the iris, **Koeppe nodules**. Adhesions of the posterior iris to the lens (**posterior synechia**) produce an irregular pupil. Thus, in iritis

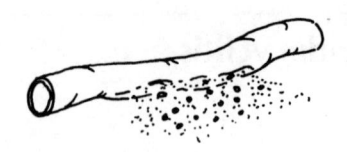

Inflamed uveal vessels leak protein and cells.

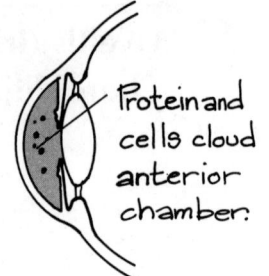

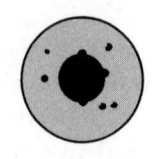

Protein and cells cloud anterior chamber.

Clumps of white cells adhere to iris.

White cell clumps adhere to posterior cornea: k.p.

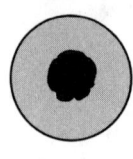

Pupil is small and irregular.

Adhesions in anterior chamber angle: anterior synechia

Iris adhered to lens: posterior synechia

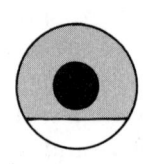

White cells in anterior chamber: hypopyon

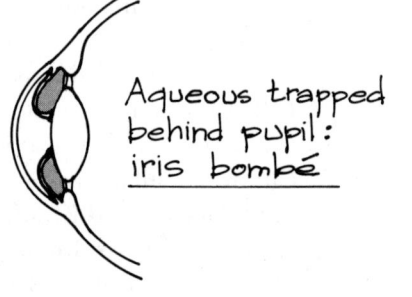

Aqueous trapped behind pupil: iris bombé

Some manifestations of uveitis (iritis)

the pupil is usually small from inflammation or irregular from posterior synechia. (*Note:* in acute glaucoma the pupil is in midposition or dilated.) If posterior synechia completely block the pupil, trapped aqueous bows the iris forward (**iris bombé**).

Adhesions in the anterior chamber angle (**anterior synechia**) may block aqueous drainage and lead to *secondary glaucoma.*

Children with Still's disease often develop iridocyclitis associated with a deposition of calcium between the corneal epithelium and Bowman's membrane, called **band keratopathy.**

Posterior Uveitis (Chorioretinitis)

Inflammatory disease of the choroid and retina is commonly caused by *toxoplasmosis, histoplasmosis,* or *toxocara* (see Chapter 14). Presumptive diagnosis is by a characteristic ophthalmoscopic appearance with some help from serologic tests. As in anterior uveitis serious loss of vision may ensue.

Granulomatous Uveitis

Granulomatous uveitis is a severe ocular inflammation with large "mutton-fat" keratic precipitates, extensive iris adhesions to the lens and in the chamber angle, and sometimes pus in the anterior chamber (*hypopyon*). Sarcoidosis, *Behçet disease, sympathetic ophthalmia,* and, less commonly, tuberculosis, syphilis, and leprosy have been implicated.

Treatment of Iritis

Topical or systemic steroids are used depending on the severity of the disease. The pupil is dilated to prevent or break posterior synechia. Immunosuppressive drugs are used in resistant cases. Mild uveitis has a good prognosis. *Secondary glaucoma* and serious loss of vision occur in severe uveitis. It is important not to treat iritis as conjunctivitis. Uveitis sometimes destroys the eye in spite of treatment.

6 Glaucoma

Open-Angle (Chronic Simple) Glaucoma

Open-angle glaucoma includes about 60% of glaucoma cases. Aqueous, produced by the ciliary body, normally flows from the *posterior* to the *anterior chamber* through the pupil, and drains through the *trabecular meshwork* and *canal of Schlemm* in the *anterior chamber angle* to veins in the sclera. In open-angle glaucoma, resistance to aqueous in the trabecular meshwork produces a rise in intraocular pressure, which gradually damages nerve fibers at the optic disc. Since there is no pain in open-angle glaucoma, serious loss of vision may occur before the diagnosis is made. The patient is usually 60 years of age or older. About 2% of the population over 40 years of age have elevated intraocular pressure on glaucoma screening tests.

Three findings are necessary for a definite diagnosis of open-angle glaucoma:

1. **Elevated intraocular pressure.** A pressure of 10-20 mm Hg is normal; 21-25 mm Hg is borderline; over 25 mm Hg is abnormal
2. **Glaucomatous cupping of the optic disc**
3. **Glaucomatous visual field loss**

Early cupping of the optic disc and visual field loss may be equivocal, even with significantly elevated intraocular pressure. For this reason there is some difference of opinion among ophthalmologists about when to begin treatment. Fortunately, open-angle glaucoma progresses slowly, so it is safe for the ophthalmologist to follow the patient carefully until the decision is made to start treatment. Once treatment is started, it usually must be continued for life.

Early in open-angle glaucoma the visual field shows peripheral nasal constriction and later a **"nasal step"** along the horizontal meridian. Without treatment the *blind spot* enlarges to form a **Seidel scotoma** and later an arcuate or **Bjerrum scotoma**. Finally, the visual field gradually constricts until only a small island of central vision remains.

Treatment is usually medical with *timolol, dipivefrin,* or *pilocarpine* eye drops and oral *carbonic anhydrase inhibitors.* In **laser trabeculoplasty,** laser burns placed in the anterior chamber angle facilitate aqueous outflow. In resistant cases a surgically created fistula allows aqueous to drain under the conjunctiva (**filtering operation; trabeculectomy**).

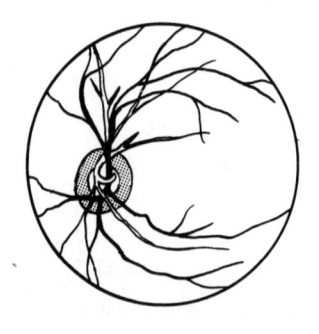

Normal optic disc 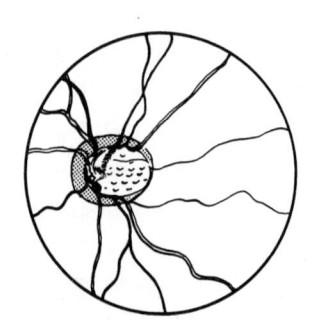   Glaucomatous cupping of optic disc

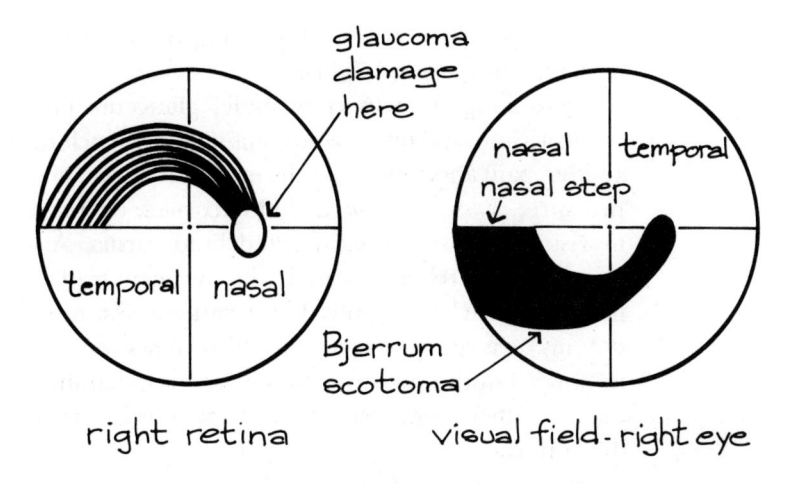

Figure: Right retina showing glaucoma damage here, temporal and nasal regions, Bjerrum scotoma. Visual field - right eye showing nasal step, nasal and temporal regions.

Typical visual field defect in chronic glaucoma reflects pattern of damaged retinal nerve fibers as they enter optic disc.

Note: Dilating the pupil for ophthalmoscopy will not induce or worsen open-angle glaucoma.

Narrow-Angle Glaucoma

Narrow-angle glaucoma accounts for about 10% of glaucoma cases. Aqueous is blocked at the anterior chamber angle before it gets to the *trabecular meshwork*. A hereditary narrow anterior chamber angle sets the stage for an acute attack. Contributing factors are hyperopia, enlargement and forward position of the crystalline lens, dilation of the pupil, and vascular congestion of the iris and ciliary body. Early symptoms include transient blurring of vision and colored halos around lights.

Acute congestive (narrow-angle) glaucoma may occur without warning. Symptoms and signs include sudden pain and redness of the eye, high intraocular pressure, *ciliary injection,* a cloudy cornea, decrease in vision, nausea, vomiting, and bradycardia. Abdominal pain from repeated vomiting may lead to inappropriate laparotomy. The treatment is **laser iridotomy or surgical iridectomy,** which allows aqueous to flow from the posterior to the anterior chamber. The chamber angle deepens and aqueous can then drain normally.

Note: (1) In acute glaucoma, the cornea is clouded: In iritis the aqueous is cloudy. (2) Dilating the pupil for ophthalmoscopy only occasionally induces narrow-angle glaucoma. If this happens, prompt treatment is curative.

Congenital Glaucoma

A cloudy infant cornea over 11 mm in diameter suggests congenital glaucoma but must be differentiated from *corneal dystrophy, mucopolysaccharidosis,* and *megalocornea.* Surgery for congenital glaucoma includes **goniotomy** and **trabeculotomy** (incising or opening the trabecular meshwork).

Secondary Glaucoma

Secondary glaucoma accounts for about 30% of glaucoma cases and can follow almost any eye disease. These include, *iridocyclitis, cataract, vascular diseases of the eye, retinal detachment, intraocular tumor,* injury, and complications of ocular surgery. *Rubeosis iridis,* a complication of diabetes and *central retinal vein occlusion,* may lead to secondary glaucoma.

Low-Tension Glaucoma

A few patients develop visual field loss and optic disc cupping even when intraocular pressure is normal. Here, optic nerve fibers at the optic disc may be abnormally vulnerable from arteriosclerotic ischemia.

Measuring Intraocular Pressure

Measure intraocular pressure as follows:

1. With the patient supine, instill a local anesthetic drop in each eye; repeat.
2. Tell the patient to look straight up. The patient's thumb may be used as a target to keep the eyes directed vertically.
3. Retract the eyelids without putting pressure on the eye. Lower the Schiøtz tonometer gently on the center of the cornea. A scale reading of 3.5 or less with the 5.5 g weight is an indication for glaucoma evaluation by an ophthalmologist. If the patient squeezes the eyelids, a false positive reading results.

7 Vascular Diseases of the Eye

Retinal Vascular Disease

The *direct ophthalmoscope* provides 15 × magnification and is of great help in diagnosing systemic vascular disease, since vascular abnormalities in the retina mirror vasculopathy elsewhere in the body.

The **reversible vascular changes in the retina** seen in essential hypertension are generalized and segmental arteriolar constriction, hemorrhages, exudates, and papilledema. These changes are also found in toxemia of pregnancy. Retinal hemorrhages and exudates suggest serious generalized vascular disease. Flame-shaped hemorrhages and cotton-wool spots (both in the nerve fiber layer close to the vitreous) are characteristic of essential hypertension with elevated diastolic blood pressure. "Blot" hemorrhages and "hard" exudates in the deeper retinal layers are suggestive of diabetic vascular disease. If essential hypertension (or toxemia) is successfully treated, the retinal abnormalities may improve. The retinal changes of diabetic retinopathy are less likely to resolve spontaneously, but may after treatment with the laser.

The **irreversible vascular changes in the retina** are generalized arteriolar narrowing, arteriovenous compression (AV nicking), and increased light reflex of the arterioles. These changes are due to permanent thickening of the vessel wall. Occasionally, when thickening is extreme, the arterioles may resemble copper or silver wire. High systolic pressure in the elderly is often associated with irreversible vessel changes. Sometimes vessel abnormalities are present when blood pressure is normal.

Hypertensive and arteriosclerotic retinal vascular disease may be graded as follows:

Grade I Early abnormalities of the retinal arterioles (narrowing, AV compression, increased light reflex)

Grade II Marked abnormalities of the retinal arterioles, suggesting significant generalized vascular disease

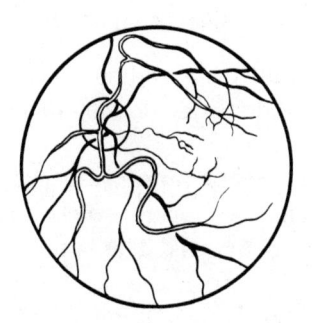

Grade II hypertensive retinopathy

Grade III Retinal hemorrhages and exudates, suggesting decompensated generalized vascular disease

Grade IV Papilledema

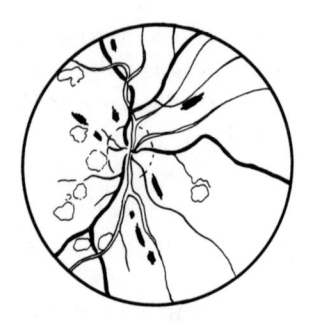

Grade III hypertensive retinopathy

Retinal Vascular Disease in Diabetes

Diabetic retinopathy is a leading cause of blindness. However, most diabetics do not develop diabetic retinopathy.

Background diabetic retinopathy is limited to the retina. Early changes include venous dilation and capillary microaneurysms. The latter are small red

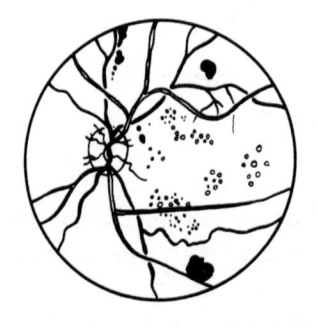

Diabetic retinopathy

dots in the fundus. Later, "blot" hemorrhages and "hard" exudates appear. Exudates and edema in the macula may cause decreased central visual acuity.

Proliferative diabetic retinopathy represents retinal neovascular proliferation occurring as a result of retinal ischemia. Abnormal vessels grow from the retina into the vitreous and may bleed. **Vitreous hemorrhage** causes sudden deterioration of vision in diabetics. Later in the disease, fibrovascular tissue in the vitreous produces *traction retinal detachment* with severe loss of vision. *Laser photocoagulation* of the retina and *vitrectomy* are effective in many cases of proliferative diabetic retinopathy.

Also associated with diabetes are the retinal vascular abnormalities of arteriosclerosis, *central* or *branch retinal vein occlusion* and neovascularization of the iris (*rubeosis iridis*) with *secondary glaucoma*.

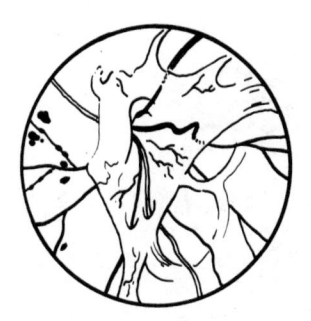

Advanced proliferative diabetic retinopathy

Central Retinal Vein Occlusion

Central retinal vein occlusion (CRVO) occurs near the lamina cribrosa of the optic nerve and is associated with hypertension, arteriosclerosis, diabetes, and various blood dyscrasias. Symptoms are rapid onset of near-total, painless loss of vision. Ophthalmoscopy reveals retinal hemorrhages and cotton-wool spots throughout the fundus with edema of the optic disc and retina. Anticoagulants or fibrinolytic agents will not restore vision. Twenty percent of patients with CRVO develop glaucoma secondary to *rubeosis iridis*.

Retinal Branch Vein Occlusion

In retinal branch vein occlusion (RBVO), only a segment of retina is involved. Complications are neovascularization of the retina or optic disc, chronic

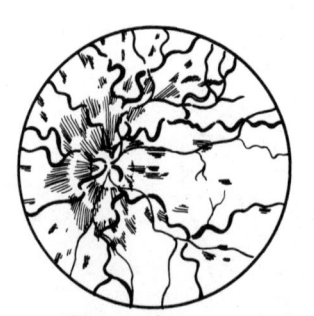

Thrombosis of central retinal vein

macular edema, and vitreous hemorrhage. Laser treatment of the abnormal new vessels or of macular edema may prevent loss of vision.

Central Retinal Artery Occlusion

Central retinal artery occlusion (CRAO) causes sudden, painless, unilateral blindness and a pale edematous retina with a cherry-red spot in the macula. As in vein occlusion, thrombosis occurs where the sclerotic artery passes through the lamina cribrosa of the optic nerve. Embolic CRAO is caused by atherosclerosis of the carotid artery in the neck. **Embolic branch retinal artery occlusion** produces a field defect corresponding to the segment of ischemic retina.

Emergency treatment of CRAO includes placement in the Trendelenburg position, rebreathing

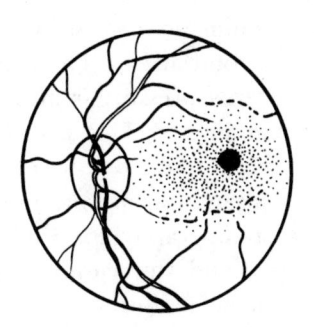

Central retinal artery occlusion

through a paper bag, massage of the eye, paracentesis of the anterior chamber, stellate ganglion block, carbonic anhydrase inhibitors, and carbon dioxide–oxygen inhalation. These maneuvers attempt to increase retinal intra-arterial pressure to dislodge the embolus to a more distal branch of the retinal artery. Prompt treatment may prevent permanent loss of vision. Drugs that interfere with platelet aggregation (such as aspirin) may make other episodes of vascular occlusion less likely.

Carotid Artery Occlusion

Suspect partial arteriosclerotic occlusion of the carotid artery in the neck in patients with **transient ischemic attacks (TIAs)**. These consist of transient ipsilateral loss of vision with contralateral weakness and paresthesias of the limbs from carotid ischemia or multiple small cerebral emboli. Between attacks the patient is asymptomatic. A bruit may be heard over the affected carotid artery. The characteristically low retinal arterial pressure is measured with an **ophthalmodynamometer**. This instrument records the pressure on the globe required to make the retinal arterioles pulsate. Carotid arteriography or digital subtraction radiography confirms the diagnosis. Timely carotid endarterectomy may prevent stroke. Untreated carotid occlusion is responsible for about 34% of strokes and has disabling sequelae similar to those of middle cerebral artery occlusion: hemiplegia, hemianesthesia, aphasia, and *homonymous hemianopsia.*

Hollenhorst plaques are small, yellow, refractile emboli at the bifurcation of retinal arterioles, caused by arteriosclerosis of the carotid artery. They suggest the danger of retinal or cerebral vascular occlusion.

Subclavian Steal Syndrome

The two subclavian arteries are circuitously connected when their vertebral artery branches join intracranially to form the basilar artery. If one subclavian artery is blocked proximal to the vertebral artery origin, the ischemic distal artery to the arm shunts blood from the sound subclavian artery, and flow in the basilar artery is reversed. Suspect this syndrome when blackouts follow arm exercise. The blood pressure is lower in the involved arm.

Occlusion of the Vertebral-Basilar Arteries

Transient basilar artery ischemia produces blurred vision, vertigo, dysarthria, dysphagia, and circumoral numbness. Hemiparesis or hemianesthesia may alternate from one side of the body to the other. "Drop attacks" occur in which the patient suddenly falls but retains consciousness. These ominous symptoms may precede a complete occlusion. Occlusion of a posterior cerebral artery produces sudden *homonymous hemianopsia* from occipital lobe infarction. Major occlusion of the vertebral-basilar arterial system produces quadriplegia and blindness, but consciousness is retained (locked-in syndrome).

Brain Stem Syndromes

Arteriosclerotic ischemia of branches of the vertebral-basilar arterial system produces various brain stem syndromes. These syndromes are caused by involvement of the cranial nerve fascicles and motor and sensory tracts in the brain stem. Tumors produce these syndromes less often.

A mnemonic for the location of the cranial nerve nuclei in the forebrain and brain stem is "2-2-4-4," indicating the cranial nerve nuclei: in the forebrain, 1 and 2; midbrain, 3 and 4; pons, 5 through 8; and medulla, 9 through 12.

The following are a few of the syndromes.

Benedikt syndrome Ischemic involvement of the red nucleus in the midbrain characterized by ipsilateral third nerve palsy with contralateral rhythmic tremor of the arm.

Weber syndrome Ipsilateral third nerve paralysis and contralateral hemiplegia resulting from a lesion in the midbrain involving the fascicle of the third cranial nerve and the corticospinal tract in the cerebral peduncle. It can also be caused by a lesion extrinsic to the brain stem.

Foville syndrome Ipsilateral sixth nerve paralysis and gaze palsy with contralateral hemiplegia caused by a pontine lesion near the sixth cranial nerve nucleus.

Wallenberg syndrome (lateral medullary syndrome) Produced by occlusion of the posterior inferior cerebellar artery or partial occlusion of the vertebral-basilar arterial system. Symptoms are vertigo, nausea, vomiting, dysphagia, dysarthria, and other symptoms from ipsilateral involvement of the 9th to 12th cranial nerve fibers in the medulla. There is contralateral impairment of pain and temperature sensation. Eye signs include nystagmus, corneal anesthesia, and oscillating (dysmetric) eye movements.

These syndromes are the result of involvement of the cranial nerve fascicle on one side (after the fibers have left the nucleus but before they exit from the brain stem) and the long motor and sensory tracts that cross below the cranial nerve nuclei. The location of the involvement accounts for the ipsilateral cranial nerve symptoms and contralateral hemiplegia ("alternating hemiplegia").

In contrast, strokes above the level of the brain stem that damage the cerebral cortex result in hemiplegia and cranial nerve signs, both of which are on the side opposite the lesion. Only cranial nerves 7 (face) and 12 (tongue) are affected, since the other cranial nerves receive innervation from both sides of the cerebral cortex.

8 Optics and Refraction

Optics

Lens strength is measured in diopters. A +1 diopter lens focuses parallel rays of light at 1 meter. Diopters and meters are inversely related; that is $D = 1/M$ or $M = 1/D$. These formulas determine the lens strength required to focus light at a certain distance and the distance at which a given lens will focus light. *Convex or "plus" lenses* converge parallel rays of light, and *concave or "minus" lenses* diverge parallel rays of light according to these formulas.

The dioptric power of the eye is 58. Substituting in the formula, $M = 1/D = 1/58 = 0.017$ meters or 17 mm. In a *schematic (or reduced) eye* the **nodal point** is 17 mm from the retina. A theoretical thin 58-diopter lens at that point would focus parallel rays of light on the retina. The eye's powerful lens system focuses parallel light rays from distant objects and, by *accommodation,* focuses divergent light rays from close objects.

Refraction

Refraction is the process of finding the combination of lenses that best corrects the patient's *myopia, hyperopia,* or *astigmatism* (**refractive error**). Like lens strength, refractive errors are measured in diopters. In **retinoscopy** a streak of light from a retinoscope is directed in the patient's eye to create a characteristic reflex. Lenses from a **trial case** are placed in a **trial frame** worn by the patient until this reflex is neutralized. This combination of lenses is close to

Optics and Refraction

the final prescription for glasses. The patient then views an eye chart while the examiner adjusts the lenses to achieve the best vision (**manifest refraction**). Instead of a trial frame a **phoropter** may be used for refraction. This is a device placed in front of the patient that permits rapid changes and combinations of lenses. For accurate refraction, especially in children, *accommodation* is paralyzed with a *cycloplegic*.

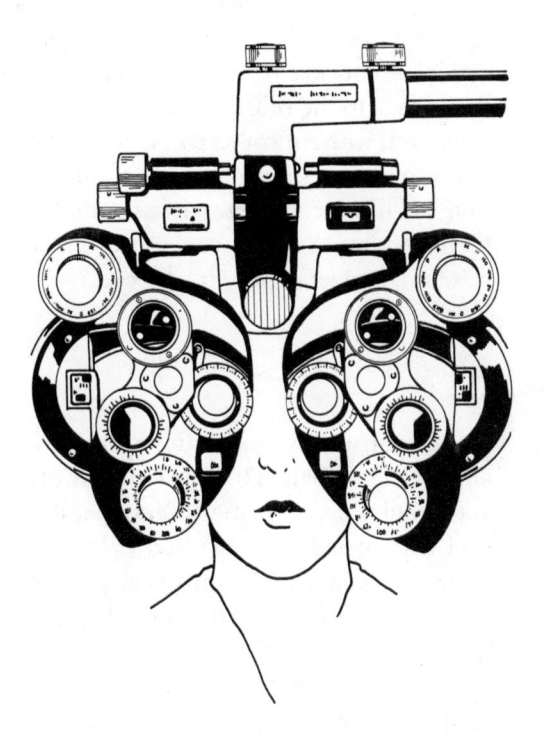

Phoropter

Emmetropia

The emmetropic eye focuses parallel rays of light on the fovea. No refractive error is present.

Myopia

The myopic eye tends to be large with a deep anterior chamber. Parallel rays of light striking the myopic eye are focused in the vitreous anterior to the retina. A concave or minus lens moves the point of focus back to the retina. The myope's distance vision is blurred without corrective lenses. The myopic eye looks smaller behind glasses. Without glasses the myopic eye has greater refractive strength than the emmetropic eye. Some myopes use this advantage to view small objects close to the eye.

Hyperopia

The hyperopic eye tends to be small with a shallow anterior chamber. The optic disc is often elevated and mimics papilledema (**pseudopapilledema**). Parallel rays of light are focused behind the retina of the hyperopic eye. A convex or **plus lens** adds refractive strength and corrects the hyperopic eye. The hyperopic eye looks enlarged behind glasses. The uncorrected hyperope must accommodate constantly to see clearly (see Accommodation below). This may cause eyestrain (*asthenopia*).

Uncorrected astigmatism

Uncorrected myopia

Uncorrected hyperopia

Emmetropia

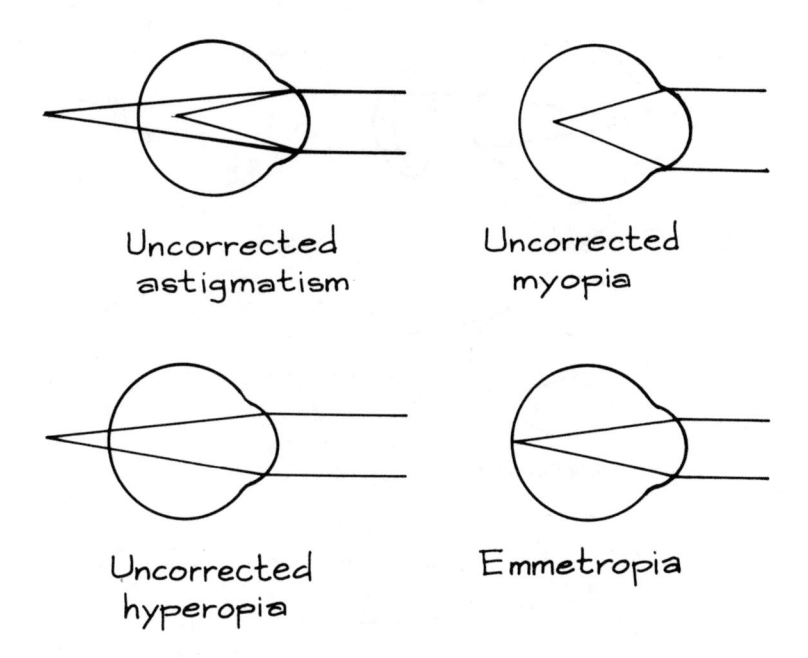

Astigmatism

The radius of curvature of the astigmatic cornea differs in different meridians. Consider a spoon where the curve along the length of the spoon is gentler than the shorter transverse curve. The cornea in astigmatism has a spoon or toric shape (**corneal astigmatism**). Similarly, the surface of the crystalline lens of the eye may have a toric shape and produce **lenticular astigmatism.** Toric (**cylindrical**) lenses with curves in different meridians, like those of a spoon, are used to correct astigmatism. The patient with uncorrected astigmatism sees vertical lines clearly and

Corrected astigmatism

Corrected myopia

Corrected hyperopia

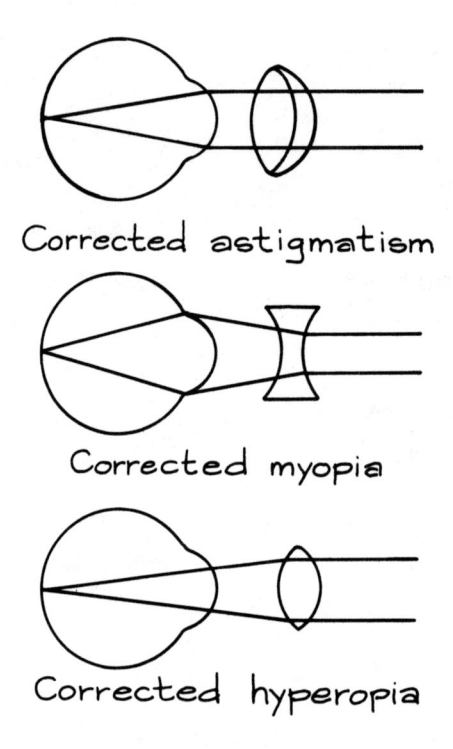

horizontal lines blurred, or vice versa, depending on the axis of the astigmatism.

Refractive Error

The refractive error (**ametropia**) of myopic, hyperopic, and astigmatic eyes is produced by variations in axial length of the eye and curvature of the cornea and lens. Long axial length, a steep curve of the cornea and lens, or both tend to produce myopia; short axial length, shallow corneal curvature, or both

Optics and Refraction 75

give rise to hyperopia. A toric surface of the cornea or lens leads to astigmatism. These factors in any combination produce the refractive error. If the predominant factor is short or long axial length rather than corneal or lens curvature, the term **axial myopia** or **axial hyperopia** is used. For example, myopia of over 4 diopters is usually axial.

Accommodation

The eye needs additional lens strength for near vision. Without accommodation, objects close to the

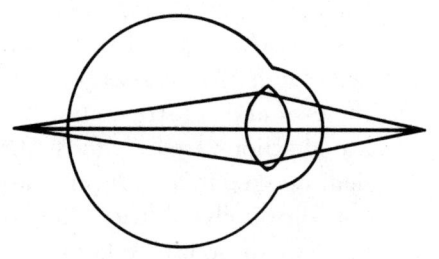

Presbyopic or unaccommodated eye

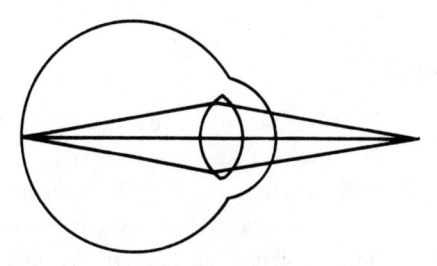

Accommodated eye

eye are focused behind the retina as in uncorrected hyperopia. In accommodation ciliary muscle contraction loosens the lens zonules, which allows the elastic lens capsule to contract, which in turn makes the lens more spherical. This increases the refractive power of the lens, which then focuses divergent rays from close objects on the retina.

Accommodation is measured by the closest distance small print can be seen. The reciprocal of this distance in meters is the **amplitude of accommodation**. Thus, accommodation, lens strength, and errors of refraction are all measured in diopters by the formula $D = 1/M$. For example, to accommodate for reading at 33 cm, 3 diopters of accommodation are necessary ($D = 1/0.33 = 3$).

Accommodation is associated with convergence of the eyes and constriction of the pupils. These associated actions are called a **synkinesis**. Thus, if a patient is asked to look from a distant object to a close one, the pupils constrict. This is the normal pupillary reaction to accommodation or the **near pupillary reflex**.

Presbyopia

With aging, the eye's ability to accommodate comfortably for reading lessens because of normal sclerosis of the lens. From about age 43 to 55, increasingly strong convex lenses are required for near vision. This normal change in the eye with age is called **presbyopia**.

Eyeglasses

Eyeglasses are prescribed to correct myopia, hyperopia, and astigmatism, Presbyopia is corrected with reading glasses or bifocals. Prisms can be ground into eyeglasses for use in *strabismus*. Protective eyeglasses prevent eye injuries from sports, tools, or machinery. Special lenses protect the eye from damage from ultraviolet, infrared, laser, and X-radiation.

Contact Lenses

Contact lenses are worn directly on the cornea by individuals who prefer contact lenses to glasses and for various medical reasons. Contact lenses are made of polymethyl methacrylate (hard lenses) or hydroxyethyl methacrylate (soft lenses). Medical indications include *aphakia, keratoconus,* and conditions requiring corneal protection.

There is a low but significant incidence of serious eye damage from contact lenses. Therefore, close professional supervision of contact lens wearers is necessary.

Ultraviolet Light

Prolonged exposure to ultraviolet light is important in the etiology of basal cell carcinoma of the skin (including the eyelids) and *pterygium*. Ultraviolet light exposure has also been implicated as a possible etiologic factor in *cataracts, macular degeneration,* and *choroidal melanoma*. Therefore, some recommend prophylactic wear of ultraviolet-blocking lenses in sunlight.

9 Strabismus

To a layman, "squint" means narrowing the eyelids, as in bright sunlight. To the ophthalmologist, squint (or strabismus) means an abnormal deviation of the eye.

Comitant Strabismus

Deviations of the eye that stay the same in all directions of gaze are **comitant**. This is in contrast to *extraocular muscle palsy*, or *incomitant strabismus*, described later in this chapter. Comitant strabismus is usually congenital, first noted in childhood, and not associated with double vision or alteration of head position. Deviation of the eye toward the nose is **esotropia**; toward the temple, **exotropia**. **Hypertropia** is an upward deviation; **hypotropia** is a downward deviation.

The eyes almost never simultaneously deviate. One eye remains straight. The brain "sees" the image of the straight eye but not that of the deviating eye, so double vision does not occur (**suppression**).

Diagnosis of Strabismus

1. Deviation of an eye is often obvious by simple observation.
2. Less obvious strabismus can be revealed by the abnormal position of the pupillary light reflex in the deviated eye when a penlight is directed into the eyes (**Hirschberg test**).

3. To accurately measure strabismus, the physician asks the patient to fixate a distant target, such as a small light, and then covers the eye that is straight (**cover-uncover test**). The deviating eye then moves to take up fixation. In *esotropia* the eye moves from a nasal position to the midline. In *exotropia* the eye moves from a temporal position to the midline. Prisms of increasing strength are placed in front of the deviating eye with the apex of the prism in the direction of the deviation until the movement is neutralized. The strength of prism required measures the strabismus in prism diopters.

A **phoria or heterophoria** (e.g., esophoria; exophoria) is a tendency for the eye to deviate. Phorias usually remain latent because of normal fusion. *Fusion* means the fovea of each eye is fixated on the same target so the individual has normal *depth perception*, or *stereopsis*. A **tropia or heterotropia** (*e.g., esotropia; exotropia*) is an abnormal deviation of an eye (*strabismus*) that makes depth perception impossible. This occurs when the tendency of the eye to deviate is so strong that fusion cannot hold the eyes straight.

Infants at any age should be referred if strabismus is suspected because untreated childhood strabismus leads to poor vision in the adult. Also, strabismus may be the first sign of a *retinoblastoma*, especially if the deviating eye has a white pupil reflex.

R L

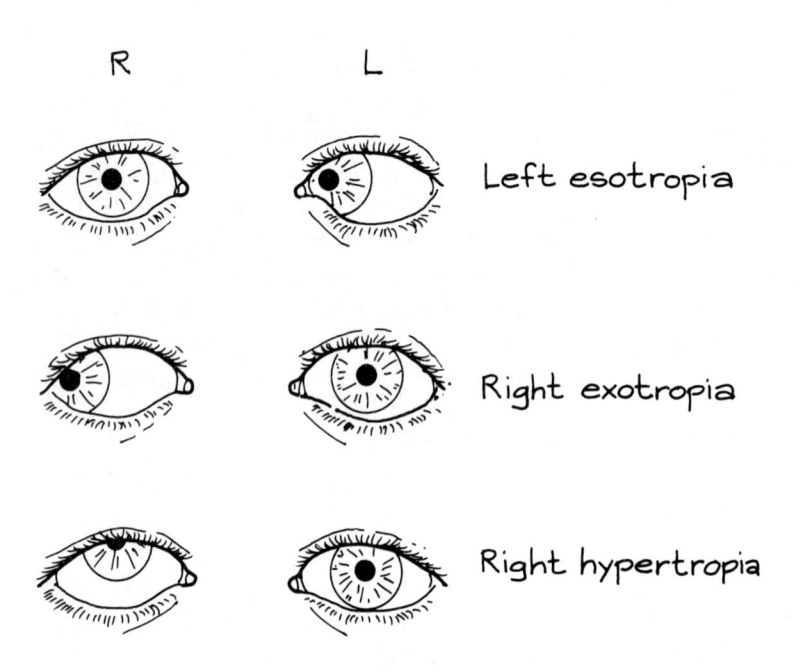

Left esotropia

Right exotropia

Right hypertropia

Esotropia

Esotropia is a defect that usually becomes manifest in infancy or early childhood.

In **alternating esotropia** first one eye crosses, then—seconds, minutes, or hours later—the other eye crosses. When one eye is crossed, the other is straight. Only the straight eye sees a clear image. *Suppression* of the image of the deviating eye prevents double vision. Alternating esotropia is compatible with the development of good vision in both eyes since the fovea of each eye is alternately stimulated while vision develops from birth to school age.

In **constant esotropia** the affected eye is crossed constantly. The other eye remains straight. The crossed eye develops **amblyopia ex anopsia** (poor vision from disuse) since the fovea of the crossed eye does not receive visual stimulation during infancy and early childhood. Untreated strabismus is a common cause of poor vision in one eye of an adult. Patching the straight eye in early childhood forces the deviated eye to fixate so it develops normal vision. Patching improves vision less as the child approaches school age. All infants should be evaluated by an ophthalmologist whenever strabismus is suspected. Surgery is often indicated for esotropia.

Accommodative esotropia occurs in hyperopic persons, who must accommodate constantly to see clearly. This accommodative effort is associated with excessive convergence because of the *synkinesis* mentioned in the section on accommodation. This extra convergence, added to the normal convergence of the eyes for near vision, results in one eye deviating toward the nose. Accommodative esotropia characteristically occurs when the patient (often a child) looks at near objects and can usually be corrected with glasses.

Exotropia

Deviation of the eye outward may be intermittent or constant in one eye or may alternate from one eye to the other. It usually occurs in late childhood or young adulthood. Surgery is often necessary. The patient is increasingly unable to converge the eyes. Normally the **near point of convergence** should be close to the nose.

Vertical Deviations

Hypertropias and hypotropias are often due to damage to the ocular nerves and muscles described in the next section. Vertical deviations may also accompany esotropia or exotropia. Vertical deviations may occur in an A or V pattern. In an A deviation, the eyes diverge in downgaze; in a V deviation, the eyes diverge in upgaze.

Extraocular Muscle Palsy (Incomitant Strabismus)

Extraocular muscle palsy (EOM palsy) should be suspected whenever a patient complains of double vision. Unlike comitant strabismus, it is acquired from damage to cranial nerves 3, 4, or 6. The cause is vascular disease (*e.g.*, hemorrhage, aneurysm, embolism, thrombosis), tumor, trauma, or infection. Deviation of the eye in EOM palsy varies with the direction of gaze and is greater when the patient tries to look in the direction of action of the palsied muscle. The patient positions the head to eliminate double vision. This position can be predicted by imagining the palsied muscle pulling on the head in the direction of its normal action.

Diseases of the ocular muscles themselves, as in

Graves' ophthalmopathy, may produce restrictive EOM palsy.

A common cause of **fourth cranial nerve** (superior oblique) palsy is trauma. The head is tilted away from the affected eye to eliminate double vision (**Bielschowsky sign**).

A common cause of **third cranial nerve palsy** with a dilated pupil (**total ophthalmoplegia**) is unruptured aneurysm of the circle of Willis. The upper eyelid is ptotic and the eye is deviated down and out. A third nerve palsy with a normal pupil (**external ophthalmoplegia**) is often associated with diabetic vascular disease.

The **sixth cranial nerve** is involved in cerebral vascular disease, diabetes, and birth trauma. The patient is unable to abduct the eye (**lateral rectus palsy**) and turns the head toward the side of the affected muscle to eliminate double vision. If sixth nerve palsy occurs without other neurologic abnormalities, the prognosis is usually good. Sixth nerve paralysis with papilledema, however, is an ominous sign of brain tumor.

Vascular disease is the most common cause of EOM palsy. Brain tumors also cause EOM palsy but are usually associated with other neurologic findings. Trauma is usually obvious from the history except when deliberately concealed, as in child abuse. Other causes of EOM palsy are infection, toxic substances, deficiency diseases, and hereditary or degenerative neurologic disease.

Double vision secondary to acquired EOM palsy

can often be relieved by appropriate surgery on the involved muscles.

Treatment of Strabismus

Objectives in treatment of strabismus are:

1. Improvement of appearance.
2. Improvement of vision (by patching or glasses).
3. The achievement of binocular vision (depth perception or stereopsis).

Surgery usually is successful in improving appearance. It is more difficult to achieve binocular vision (depth perception or stereopsis) although some degree of fusion is often attained. Children often seem to have better coordination after strabismus surgery.

Orthoptics

Orthoptics includes techniques of examination and treatment of strabismus by a trained **orthoptist** under the supervision of an ophthalmologist. The orthoptist uses an **amblyoscope,** an instrument with lighted tubes moved horizontally and vertically, which project an image on the fovea of each eye, to measure and stimulate fusion. **Fusion** occurs when the brain perceives the two images as one (**binocular vision**). There are increasing grades of binocular vision leading to normal **stereopsis** or **depth perception.**

10 Cataract

Any opacity in the lens of the eye is a cataract. Cataracts are best seen after dilatation of the pupil. Look through the +5 lens of the ophthalmoscope about 6 inches from the patient. You will see a black silhouette of the cataract against the background of the red pupil reflex. Slit lamp examination reveals details of the lens changes. Three common cataract types are:

Cortical—Spokelike opacities project centrally from the periphery of the lens.
Nuclear—The center of the lens develops increasing yellow-brown discoloration.
Posterior subcapsular—An opacity is located in the center of the back of the lens just under the posterior capsule.

Cataract removal ranks among the most frequently performed surgical operations. Visual acuity is usually 20/60 or worse, but the main indication for surgery is when loss of vision interferes with normal daily activities.

Intracapsular cataract extraction involves the removal of the entire lens with its capsule. This procedure is done less often than extracapsular cataract extraction.

Extracapsular cataract extraction is the preferred method of cataract extraction. It can be visualized by comparing the lens of the eye to a grape. The skin of the grape is opened and its anterior portion (anterior lens capsule) is removed. The contents of the grape (nucleus and cortex) are then removed.

Cortical   Nuclear Sclerosis

Posterior Subcapsular   Mature

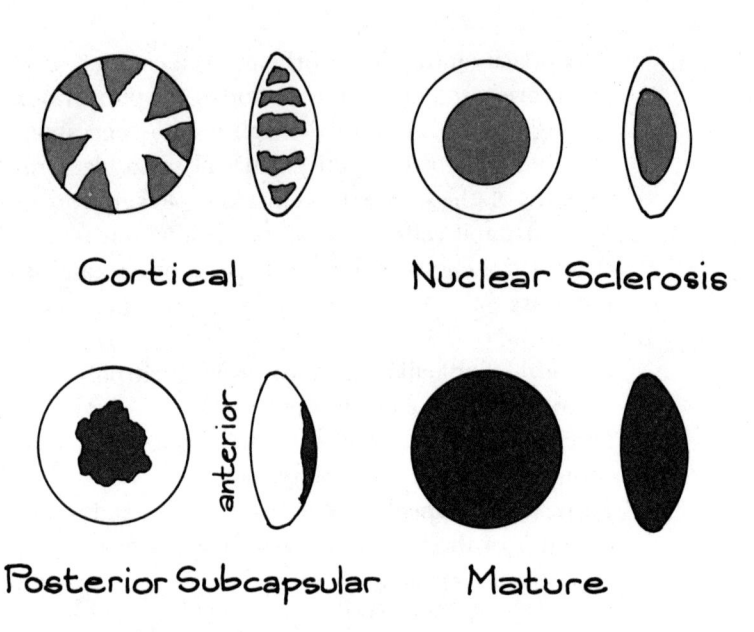

Common Cataract Types

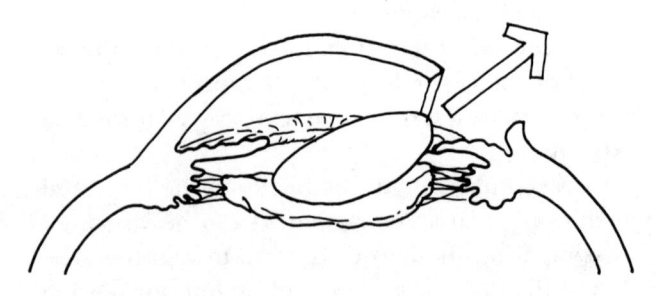

Extracapsular cataract extraction

The posterior skin of the grape (posterior lens capsule) is left in the eye. This intact posterior lens capsule holds the vitreous in its normal position and thus makes postoperative *cystoid macular edema, secondary glaucoma,* and *retinal detachment* less likely than after intracapsular cataract extraction.

Skill is required to avoid serious technical problems in cataract surgery. The operating microscope, special instruments, fine sutures, and constantly improving techniques make cataract extraction a precise, safe procedure.

In children, cataracts are usually congenital or traumatic. Maternal rubella in the first trimester of pregnancy is a cause of congenital cataract. These children may also have deafness, mental retardation, and cardiovascular defects. A congenital cataract that produces severe loss of vision is treated by extracapsular cataract surgery.

If the posterior lens capsule becomes cloudy after extracapsular surgery in children or adults, it must be opened surgically (**discission**) or with the laser (**laser capsulotomy**).

Complications occur after cataract surgery in about 5% of cases, and occasionally an eye becomes blind.

After cataract extraction, unless an *intraocular lens* is implanted, thick glasses or contact lenses must be worn since surgical removal of the cataractous lens results in a high degree of hyperopia. Thick cataract glasses are hard for patients to get used to, since everything looks magnified and side vision is reduced.

Intraocular lenses (IOL) are placed in the eye at

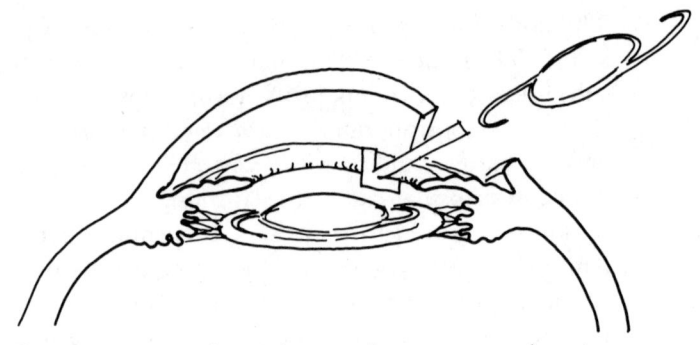

Posterior chamber lens implant

the time of cataract extraction in most older patients. There is some risk with IOL implantation in children and young adults, since the long-term effects of various IOLs inside the eye are not known. Lens implants are popular because patients have good vision without thick glasses or contact lenses. However, lens implants carry some risk of early or late complications. Indications, techniques, and intraocular lens composition and design are constantly being modified.

11 Neuro-Ophthalmology

Many central nervous system diseases have ocular manifestations. A few selected topics in neuro-ophthalmology are included here. The section on *extraocular muscle palsy* in Chapter 9 should be reviewed.

Miosis

Miosis (pupillary constriction) is normal in infancy and old age. It is induced by bright light, sleep, and accommodation. Other causes are *Horner syndrome*, the *Argyll Robertson pupil*, pilocarpine treatment of glaucoma, coma, narcotic intoxication, *iritis*, and some pontine lesions.

Mydriasis

The most common cause of mydriasis (pupillary dilatation; *internal ophthalmoplegia*) is accidental or intentional instillation of atropine or an atropine-like chemical into the eye. Pilocarpine has no effect on a pupil dilated as the result of a pharmacologic agent. If the cause of the dilatation is neurologic (interruption of the parasympathetic fibers in cranial nerve 3), pilocarpine constricts the pupil. Mydriasis is seen in epidural or subdural hematoma, *acute glaucoma*, contusion of the globe, and deep anesthesia, and can be a sign of death. The pupil is dilated in dim light, excitement, and youth. Mydriasis is also seen in *Adie's pupil* and *total ophthalmoplegia*. The pupil of a blind eye is usually not dilated since the consensual pupillary reflex from the sound eye maintains normal

Basic Ophthalmology

right   left

(•)   (●)

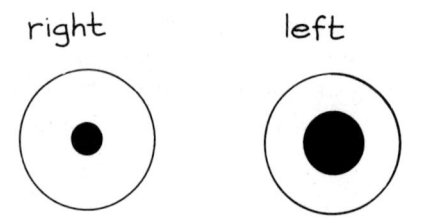

Mydriasis left; right pupil normal
Miosis right; left pupil normal
Horner's pupil, right
Adies' pupil, left
Pilocarpine in right eye (or any miotic)
Tropicamide in left eye (or any mydriatic)
Third cranial nerve lesion, left
Light directed in right eye
Iritis, right eye
Acute glaucoma, left eye

   Anisocoria — possible causes

pupil size. Physiologic *anisocoria* is a normal variant in about 20% of the population.

Nystagmus

Involuntary oscillating horizontal, vertical, or rotatory eye movements can be congenital or due to CNS, cerebellar, labryinthine, or vestibular disease. Nystagmus also occurs in gaze weakness from any cause.

Disassociated nystagmus Nystagmus in which the movements in the two eyes are dissimilar, as in multiple sclerosis.
End-position nystagmus Normal in extreme right or left gaze.
Jerk nystagmus A fast movement in one direction with a slow movement in the other. It is named from the direction of the fast component.
Vestibular nystagmus Nystagmus due to vestibular disturbance. Examples are the jerk nystagmus of *multiple sclerosis*, Meniere's disease, *Wallenberg syndrome*, and cerebellar disease.
Latent nystagmus Nystagmus that occurs in one eye when the other eye is covered. It can be an isolated finding or be associated with *strabismus*.
Pendular nystagmus Nystagmus in which there are equal oscillations in both directions. The condition occurs in infants and children with poor vision.
Railroad or optokinetic nystagmus The normal nystagmus occurring when looking out from a moving train or at a rotating *optokinetic drum*. It is present in feigned blindness and absent in blindness and parietal-lobe brain tumors.

Horner Syndrome

Normally, the vertical height of the palpebral fissure and pupil size are regulated by the autonomic nervous system. Decreased sympathetic stimulation to

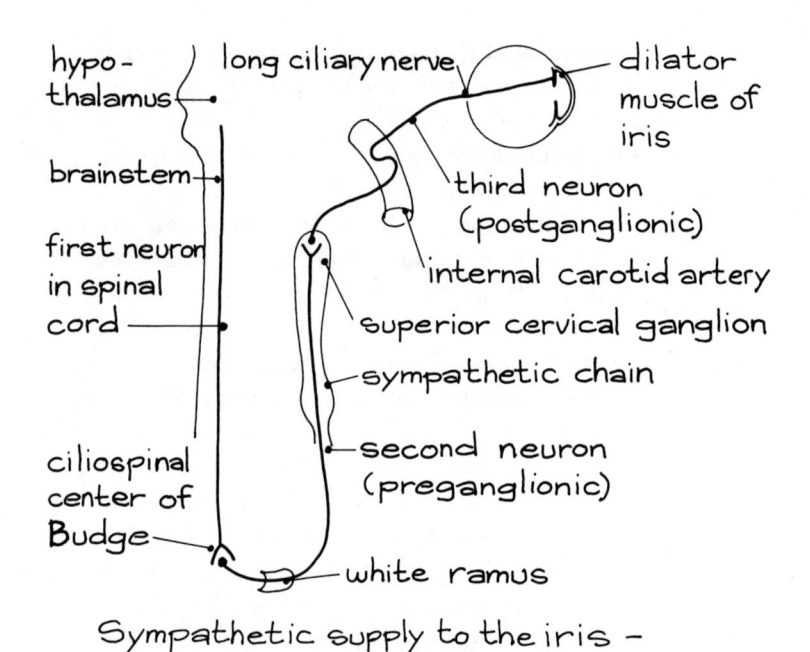

```
hypo-          long ciliary nerve              dilator
thalamus                                       muscle of
                                               iris
brainstem
                             third neuron
first neuron                 (postganglionic)
in spinal                    internal carotid artery
cord                         superior cervical ganglion
                             sympathetic chain

                             second neuron
ciliospinal                  (preganglionic)
center of
Budge
                             white ramus
```

Sympathetic supply to the iris –
Interruption causes Horner syndrome

the smooth muscle of the eyelids and iris results in Horner syndrome with ptosis, miosis, and sometimes ipsilateral absence of sweating. Horner syndrome is caused by lesions anywhere in the sympathetic pathway that goes from the hypothalamus to the brain stem and upper spinal cord (**first neuron**); then to the cervical sympathetic chain and superior cervical ganglion (**second neuron**); and finally, via the carotid plexus, first division of the fifth cranial nerve, and long ciliary nerve, to the iris (**third neuron**). Horner syndrome may be congenital, inflammatory, neoplastic, traumatic, or idiopathic. The Horner pupil dilates less than the normal pupil in darkness. The normal pupil dilates with cocaine and hydroxyamphetamine. Failure of a miotic pupil to dilate with cocaine indicates Horner syndrome from a second-neuron (preganglionic) or third-neuron (postganglionic) lesion. Dilation with hydroxyamphetamine and not with cocaine indicates a second-neuron lesion. Third-neuron lesions usually have a good prognosis (*e.g.*, *Raeder* and *Horton syndromes*). Second-neuron lesions may be associated with advanced breast or lung cancer.

Migraine

Eye symptoms are important in migraine. Typically the patient complains of a bilateral defect in central vision with a surrounding bright shimmering border (**scintillating scotoma**). Whereas the unilateral blurring of vision in carotid occlusive disease lasts a few seconds or minutes, the scotoma of migraine lasts about 20 minutes. This is usually followed by a severe headache with nausea. In severe forms hemianopsias, cranial nerve palsies, and hemiplegia occur. There are many variations of migraine. Ergotamine tartrate 0.5 mg IM will often abort an attack and establish the diagnosis. Propranolol may be useful for treatment.

Optic Neuritis

Optic neuritis is an inflammation either at the optic disc (**papillitis**) or in the part of the optic nerve behind the globe of the eye (**retrobulbar neuritis**). Symptoms are unilateral loss of vision, pain on movement of the globe, and a central scotoma. Vision usually improves in a few weeks. In retrobulbar neuritis the fundus looks normal. Papillitis, which mimics papilledema, produces early loss of vision. In papilledema, any loss of vision occurs late in the disease. This helps differentiate the two conditions. Furthermore, papilledema is usually bilateral whereas papillitis is usually unilateral.

Weeks or months after the onset of optic neuritis the optic disc often becomes pale temporally. A completely white optic disc is characteristic of **optic atrophy**.

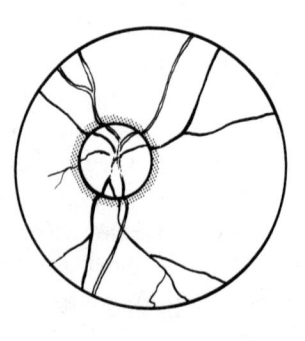

Optic atrophy

In the "swinging flashlight test," a penlight is passed from one pupil to the other. The normal pupil constricts slightly the instant the light strikes it. If slight dilatation occurs, the **Marcus Gunn pupillary reaction** is present. This reaction, which is also called an **afferent pupillary defect,** is a sensitive sign of optic neuritis and other diseases affecting afferent conduction in the optic nerve.

Optic neuritis may be misdiagnosed in the presence of an unsuspected brain tumor, such as *meningioma of the tuberculum sellae.*

The etiology of optic neuritis is unknown in most cases. About 20% of patients develop multiple sclerosis. Do not discuss this possibility, however, since the patient may become unnecessarily depressed. Although vision in optic neuritis usually improves without treatment, ACTH or systemic steroid medication is often given.

Other causes of optic neuritis or optic atrophy are infection, hereditary disease, vascular occlusion, tumors, trauma, and glaucoma.

Anterior Ischemic Optic Neuropathy

Anterior ischemic optic neuropathy (AION) is an ischemic infarct of the optic nerve at or near the lamina cribrosa. Typically, a person over 60 years of age with vascular disease develops sudden unilateral loss of vision, an *altitudinal visual field defect* (usually the lower half of the visual field) and segmental swelling and hemorrhage of the optic disc. Color vision is abnormal and an *afferent pupillary defect* is present. Unlike *temporal arteritis* (discussed below), the sedimentation rate is 40 or less and steroid medication has no effect. The visual prognosis is poor. Optic atrophy occurs after the optic disc swelling subsides. The second eye is affected months or years later in one-third of patients, leading to a pseudo–Foster Kennedy syndrome (optic atrophy on one side and disc edema on the other, without brain tumor).

Retrobulbar (or posterior) ischemic optic neuropathy is much less common than AION but does occur in some instances.

Cranial (Temporal) Arteritis

Temporal arteritis is a form of AION that is less common than the non-arteritic form discussed above. It occurs in patients in their late 60s or older. Premonitory visual symptoms are followed by more severe loss of vision than in non-arteritic AION. The optic disc is normal or swollen. Occasionally the clinical picture is that of central retinal artery occlusion. Malaise, fever, weight loss, polymyalgia, head pain, and pain with chewing are associated findings. The sedimentation rate is over 50. Biopsy of the involved temporal artery shows giant-cell arteritis. Systemic steroids should be given if the diagnosis is suspected, since dramatic improvement in vision may follow. Without treatment, severe loss of vision is likely. In

75% of untreated patients, the second eye is involved later.

Papilledema

Papilledema classically means bilateral edema of the optic nerve heads caused by increased intracranial pressure. Hemorrhages occur on or near the swollen disc. Retinal venous pulsation, when present, rules out papilledema. Optic nerve head edema is also seen in *hypotony, orbital tumors,* hypertension, meningitis, and severe anemia. In papilledema central vision remains normal until late in the disease, in contrast to *papillitis,* in which there is early loss of central vision. This is important since the two conditions look similar on ophthalmoscopic examination.

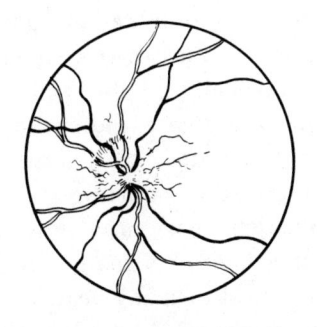

Early papilledema

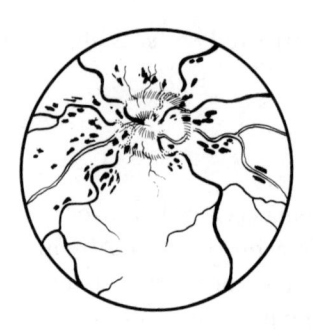

Advanced papilledema

Multiple Sclerosis (MS)

Demyelinization of the CNS of unknown etiology produces variable symptoms including paresthesias and weakness of the legs and arms, ataxia, and emotional disturbances. Common eye signs are *optic neuritis* and internuclear ophthalmoplegia. **Internuclear ophthalmoplegia** is due to involvement of the medial longitudinal fasciculus in the brain stem. On attempted right or left gaze, there is ipsilateral paralysis of the medial rectus muscle of the adducting eye and nystagmus of the abducting eye.

Some MS patients have progressive disability and become incapacitated, but many have lesser symptoms over a period of many years. The classic but infrequent **Charcot's triad** includes nystagmus, scanning speech, and intention tremor.

Brain Tumors

Eye symptoms and signs are present in about 60% of patients with brain tumors. Generalized symptoms include bilateral papilledema, headache, sixth nerve palsy, and a fixed dilated pupil. Some localizing signs are as follows:

Frontal lobe tumors can cause personality changes and unilateral optic atrophy with contralateral

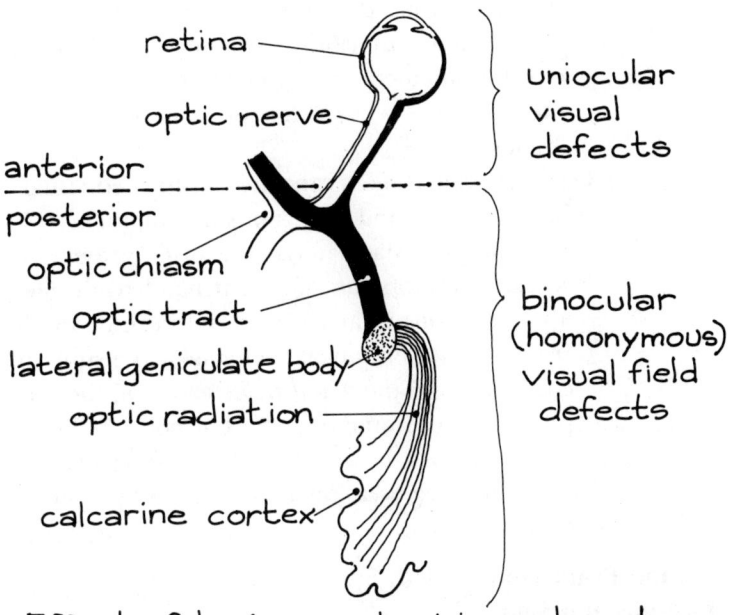

[Diagram showing:
- retina
- optic nerve
- anterior
- posterior
- optic chiasm
- optic tract
- lateral geniculate body
- optic radiation
- calcarine cortex

With brackets indicating:
- uniocular visual defects (anterior structures)
- binocular (homonymous) visual field defects (posterior structures)]

Effect of lesions anterior and posterior to the optic chiasm.

papilledema (**Foster Kennedy syndrome**). Some frontal lobe tumors are "silent."

Temporal lobe tumors can cause olfactory, gustatory, and formed visual hallucinations with incongruous superior quadrantic homonymous hemianopsia ("pie-in-sky") due to damage to the visual radiation in Meyer's loop.

Parietal lobe tumors cause difficulty in reading, writing, and arithmetic (alexia, agraphia, and acalculia). These signs with right homonymous hemianopsia constitute the **Gerstmann syndrome**, which indicates dominant parietal lobe involvement. Inferior quadrantopsia with reduced optokinetic nystagmus to the side opposite the lesion is characteristic of parietal lobe lesions.

Occipital lobe tumors can cause unformed visual hallucinations and congruous homonomous hemianopsia. Macular vision is often preserved.

Brain stem tumors can cause **Parinaud syndrome**, a paralysis of upward gaze in both eyes, typically from a midbrain pineal tumor near the superior colliculi. As in the *Argyll Robertson pupil*, the pupils react to accommodation, but not to light.

The vascular *brain stem syndromes* discussed in Chapter 7 are occasionally produced by brain stem tumors.

Common Brain Tumors with Eye Symptoms and Signs

Glioblastoma multiforme of the adult usually causes generalized CNS symptoms, such as seizures and

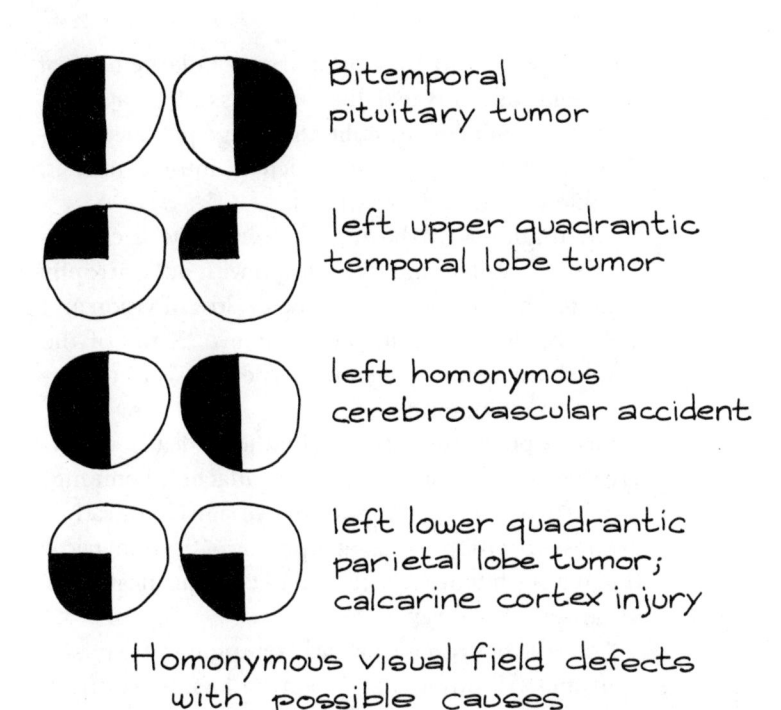

Bitemporal pituitary tumor

left upper quadrantic temporal lobe tumor

left homonymous cerebrovascular accident

left lower quadrantic parietal lobe tumor; calcarine cortex injury

Homonymous visual field defects with possible causes

personality changes, that progress to drowsiness and coma. The localizing signs listed above may help in diagnosis.

Cerebellar medulloblastoma of childhood leads to generalized symptoms of increased intracranial pressure: headache, vomiting, papilledema, and sixth nerve palsy.

Pituitary adenoma results in loss of vision, optic atrophy, and classical bitemporal hemianopsia. Impotence, amenorrhea, and other hormone imbalances are due to hypopituitarism. Enlargement of the sella turcica is usually seen on skull X-ray.

Meningioma of the sphenoid ridge produces unilateral exophthalmos, extraocular muscle paresis, double vision, and loss of vision.

Meningioma of the tuberculum sellae is characterized by unilateral loss of vision with optic atrophy that may mimic *optic neuritis*. Later, loss of vision and field changes occur in the other eye. X-ray of the skull characteristically shows hyperostosis in the region of meningiomas.

Craniopharyngioma in childhood leads to increased intracranial pressure, headaches, vomiting, and hydrocephalus. Important eye signs in the adult are loss of vision, optic atrophy, and asymmetrical fluctuating bitemporal field defects. Calcification is often seen on X-ray.

Acoustic neuroma The early symptoms of acoustic neuroma are tinnitus and hearing loss. Since these symptoms are common in patients without tumors, eye symptoms help in diagnosis. Decreased corneal sensation is caused by disturbance of the fifth cranial nerve. Irritability of the seventh cranial nerve is manifested by twitching of the eyelid.

12 Eyelid, Lacrimal, and Orbital Diseases and Surgery

Ophthalmic plastic and reconstructive surgery includes operations on the eyelids, lacrimal system, and orbit.

Eyelids

The eyelids must be properly positioned and functioning to maintain the tear film that keeps the surface of the cornea and conjunctiva moist and protects the eye. Abnormalities of the eyelids may lead to keratitis, corneal vascularization, and, in extreme cases, destruction of the eye. Surgery is done to correct eyelid malpositions, including *blepharoptosis, entropion, ectropion, eyelid retraction, blepharochalasis, trichiasis, symblepharon, lagophthalmos,* eyebrow ptosis, and traumatic and congenital deformities.

Blepharoptosis

The position of the upper eyelid is controlled by the levator palpebrae superioris muscle, supplied by the third nerve, and Müller's muscle, supplied by sympathetic nerves. Ptosis (drooping of the upper eyelid) results from abnormalities of these nerves or muscles. In children, ptosis is usually congenital. Most adult ptosis is due to stretching or disinsertion of the levator aponeurosis. Ptosis is also associated with *Horner syndrome, third cranial nerve palsy,* myasthenia gravis, muscular dystrophy, myotonic dystrophy, and injuries and may follow operations on the eye and adnexa. Surgical correction of ptosis requires a detailed knowledge of upper eyelid anatomy.

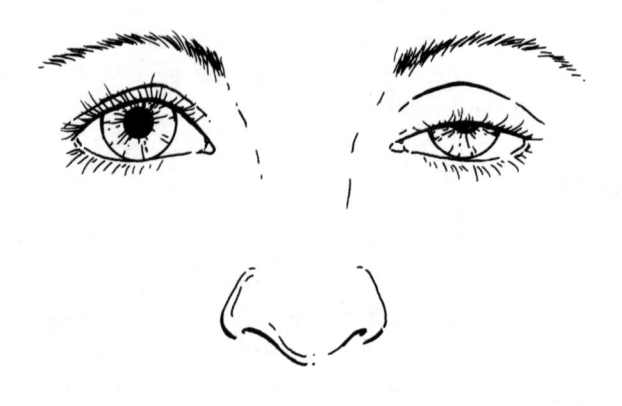

Blepharoptosis

Eyelid Tumors

In the child, the **capillary hemangioma** appears as a circumscribed dark-red mass anywhere on the eyelids or face. It usually regresses spontaneously or after injection with steroid.

In the adult, **basal cell carcinoma** of the eyelids is common in persons with long exposure to sunlight. **Squamous carcinoma** is less common but more aggressive. Both are treated by surgical excision with frozen section control. Neglected lesions can invade the orbit and destroy the eye. *Mohs fresh-tissue surgery* by a dermatologist trained in this technique, followed by surgical reconstruction, is useful for advanced lesions.

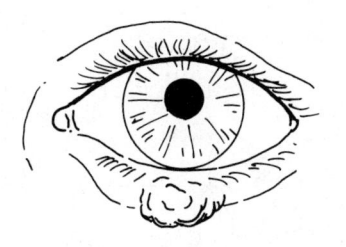

Basal or squamous cell
eyelid carcinoma

Lacrimal System

The lacrimal gland and accessory glands in the eyelids secrete mucus, tears, and oil, which make up the tear film that lubricates and protects the conjunctiva and cornea. Tears drain through the lacrimal puncta and canaliculi to the lacrimal sac and nasolacrimal duct to empty under the inferior turbinate into the nose. Any part of this system can be obstructed by congenital defects, infection, or injury.

Lacrimal Obstruction

Symptoms of lacrimal obstruction include tearing, "mattering," a discharge from the inner corner of the eye, and sometimes a mass in the region of the lacrimal sac. Pressure on this mass often forces mucus or pus out of the lacrimal puncta. Recurrent *dacryocystitis* is commonly associated with lacrimal obstruction.

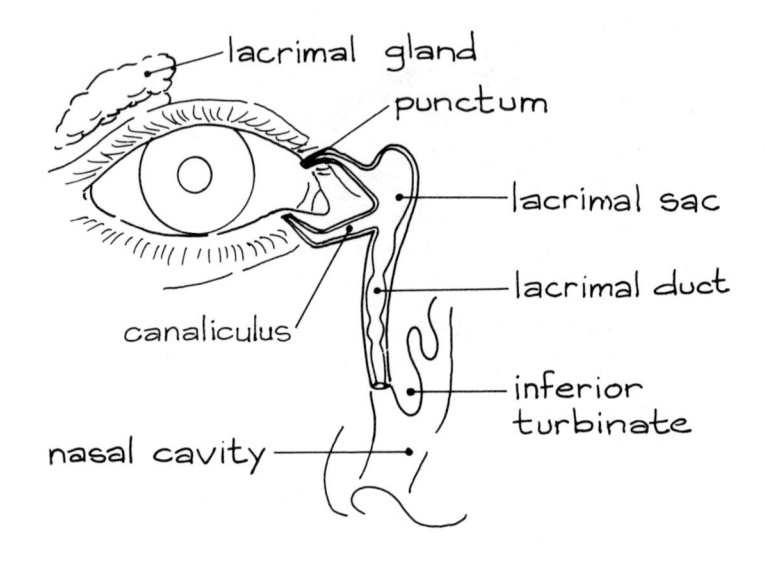

Lacrimal drainage system

Probing of the Nasolacrimal Duct

Persistent lacrimal obstruction in infants usually responds to probing of the nasolacrimal duct. Probing in adults is less likely to relieve obstruction.

Silicone Intubation

Silicone tubing swaged onto metal cannulas is passed, via the puncta, through the lacrimal drainage system to the nose, where the ends are tied just inside the nostril. This makes a complete loop that acts as a stent in the treatment of childhood and adult obstruction and after repair of canalicular injuries.

Dacryocystorhinostomy (DCR)

Persistent lacrimal obstruction at or distal to the lacrimal sac is treated by surgically creating a fistula from the lacrimal sac to the nose through a hole created in the bone between the lacrimal sac and nasal cavity.

Conjunctivodacryocystorhinostomy (CDCR)

Congenital, inflammatory, or traumatic obstruction of the lacrimal canaliculi is treated by placing a small Pyrex glass (Jones) tube from the inner corner of the eye to the nasal cavity through a hole in the adjacent bone.

Overproduction of Tears

Almost any eye disease may be associated with tearing from eye irritation. This is usually bilateral, in contrast to the unilateral tearing of mechanical obstruction. Tearing from eye irritation is not an indication for surgery (DCR or CDCR).

Ocular Tumors
Retinoblastoma

Retinoblastoma should be suspected in a child with a white pupil and strabismus. This is the common malignant intraocular tumor of childhood. It is characteristically multicentric and is transmitted as a dominant trait in bilateral cases. Calcification is an important X-ray finding. Retinoblastoma is similar to childhood neuroblastoma in histology and radiosensitivity. Survival is related to early diagnosis and prompt treatment. Advanced lesions require enucleation. Cryotherapy or radiation may control smaller tumors. Survivors who marry should have genetic counseling.

Choroidal Melanoma

Choroidal melanoma is the common adult intraocular malignant tumor. Small asymptomatic melanomas are found on routine eye examination. Large tumors produce loss of vision, intraocular inflammation, hemorrhage, or *secondary glaucoma*. A smooth blue-grey or brown elevation of the retina is seen with the ophthalmoscope. The tumor is less malignant than the malignant melanoma of the skin. Small or doubtful tumors are kept under observation, photocoagulated, or treated with radiation. Large tumors require enucleation.

Orbital Diseases

Exophthalmos

Exophthalmos or **proptosis** is unilateral or bilateral protrusion of the eye(s), most commonly from thyroid disease. Exophthalmos can also be caused by

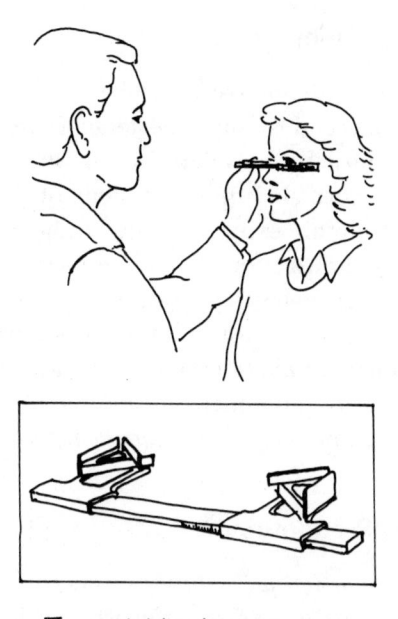

Exophthalmometry

orbital pseudotumor and by benign and malignant orbital tumors.

Proptosis is measured with an **exophthalmometer**. This is a mirrored device placed against the lateral orbital rims that projects an image of each cornea on a millimeter scale read by the examiner. Normally the cornea is 10 mm to 20 mm anterior to the lateral orbital rim. A distance of over 20 mm is considered to be beginning proptosis; 25 mm to 30 mm is marked proptosis. *CT scan* and *ultrasound* studies are indicated in most patients with exophthalmos.

Thyroid Ophthalmopathy

Thyroid ophthalmopathy is the most common cause of proptosis and is usually bilateral. Thyroid (Graves') disease must be considered even when all thyroid tests are normal. Important signs of thyroid ophthalmopathy are exophthalmos, lid lag on downgaze, and eyelid retraction. Eyelid retraction in thyroid disease exaggerates the appearance of proptosis. The ocular muscles and orbital tissues become inflamed and swollen. Limitation of upward gaze and diplopia are common. Treatment includes systemic steroids and sometimes *orbital decompression*.

Orbital Pseudotumor

The term *orbital pseudotumor* refers to a number of inflammatory processes in the orbit, such as myositis, pseudolymphoma, and granulomatous inflamma-

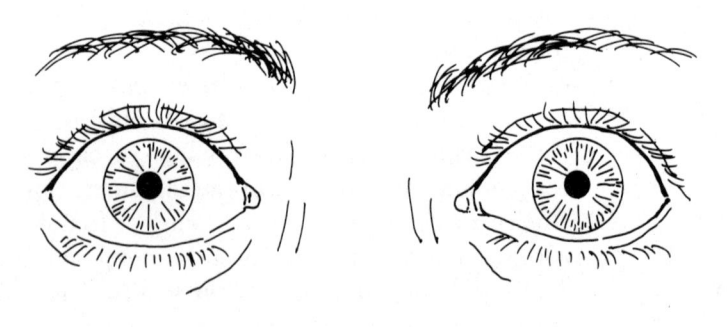

Graves' disease

tion. In these conditions, unlike thyroid ophthalmopathy, proptosis is usually unilateral. Biopsy may be necessary for diagnosis. Proptosis, secondary oculomotor paralysis with diplopia, and loss of vision from orbital pseudotumor may regress, persist, or progress after treatment with systemic steroids.

Orbital Tumors

Cavernous Hemangioma

Cavernous hemangioma is the most common adult orbital neoplasm and the most amenable to surgery. It causes painless proptosis.

Mucocele

Mucoceles erode from the adjacent frontal or ethmoid sinus into the orbit and produce secondary proptosis. Surgery is curative.

Dermoid Cyst

In children, a dermoid cyst is usually superficial and easily excised. In adults it may involve the orbit, an adjacent sinus, the temporal fossa, the cranium, or the skin surface, so excision can be difficult.

Meningioma

Intracranial *meningiomas of the sphenoidal ridge and tuberculum sellae* can involve the optic nerve or extend to the orbit to produce loss of vision and proptosis (see Chapter 11). **Primary intraorbital meningiomas** also cause proptosis. They are benign, slow-growing tumors usually closely applied to the optic nerve. Surgical excision is likely to destroy vision.

Optic Nerve Glioma

Optic nerve glioma is a benign, hamartomatous tumor that typically appears in preschool children, causing loss of vision, and is often associated with neurofibromatosis. Symptoms and signs depend on the location of the tumor: in the orbit, proptosis; in the optic canal, enlargement visible on X-ray; intracranially, pituitary and hypothalamic disorders with increased intracranial pressure. Surgery is done for diagnosis, marked proptosis, or elevated intracranial pressure.

Mixed Tumor of the Lacrimal Gland

Mixed tumor of the lacrimal gland is a benign tumor but tends to recur after surgery. Late malignant change is not uncommon.

Adenoid Cystic Carcinoma of the Lacrimal Gland

This malignant tumor has a poor prognosis even with radical surgery and chemotherapy. Symptoms are proptosis and pain. X-ray shows bone erosion in the lacrimal fossa.

Rhabdomyosarcoma

Rhabdomyosarcoma is the most common primary malignant orbital tumor in children. It causes rapid, progressive proptosis. It is treated with radiation and chemotherapy but has a poor prognosis.

Lymphomas of the Orbit

Lymphomas of the orbit may be primary in the orbit but are usually associated with lymphoid malignancy elsewhere. Proptosis and a salmon-red growth in the conjunctival fornix occur. Treatment is by radiation.

Secondary Orbital Tumors

The orbit may be invaded by tumors of the eye (*retinoblastoma, melanoma*). It may also be invaded by tumors of the conjunctiva and eyelids (basal and squamous carcinoma, melanoma) as well as carcinomas from the paranasal sinuses, nasopharynx, lacrimal sac, and cranial cavity.

Metastatic Tumors

Metastatic tumors characteristically infiltrate the choroid inside the eye of the adult but involve the extraocular soft tissues of the orbit in the child.

In the adult, metastatic tumors from the lung or prostate in the male and the breast in the female infiltrate and elevate the choroid and may be mistaken for a retinal detachment.

Less commonly in the adult, metastatic tumors may involve the extraocular orbital soft tissue and produce *exophthalmos,* pain, double vision, and loss of vision. Metastatic breast cancer may be associated with *enophthalmos.*

In the child, metastatic tumors invade the orbit rather than the eye itself. The most common type is the **metastatic neuroblastoma from the adrenal gland.** This tumor is suspected when proptosis in a child is associated with eyelid ecchymosis.

Orbital Surgery

An anterior or lateral (Kronlein) orbitotomy is done for biopsy or removal of orbital tumors. Loss of vision, blepharoptosis, and extraocular muscle paralysis (with double vision) are possible after any orbital operation.

Thyroid ophthalmopathy is treated by **orbital decompression** when visual loss is threatened or for extreme proptosis. The floor and one or more walls of the orbit are removed to allow more space for swollen orbital tissues.

Orbital floor fractures are repaired through a lower eyelid incision or a Caldwell-Luc antrotomy.

Orbital reconstruction is done for inability to wear an artificial eye.

13 The Cornea

Corneal injury and inflammation are described in Chapter 4. Diseases of the cornea include corneal dysgeneses, dystrophies, and degenerations.

Corneal Dysgeneses

Corneal dysgeneses are genetic structural abnormalities of the cornea: **microcornea** (small cornea); **cornea plana** (flat cornea); **megalocornea** (large cornea); **keratoglobus** (large, thin cornea); and **sclerocornea** (the sclera extends into the cornea).

Corneal Dystrophies

Corneal dystrophies are familial, multiple corneal opacities described by their appearance (ringlike, macular, granular, lattice, crystalline, guttata, etc.) or by eponyms (Meesman, Cogan, Reis-Buckler, Groenouw, Biber, Schnyder, Fuchs, etc).

Corneal Degenerations

Corneal degenerations are associated with **previous inflammation** (amyloid degeneration, Salzmann nodular degeneration, lipid degeneration); **geographic factors** (spheroidal degeneration, keratinoid degeneration, Labrador keratopathy, actinic keratopathy); or are **marginal degenerations of uncertain etiology** (Terrien marginal degeneration, Mooren ulcer, pellucid marginal degeneration, furrow degeneration).

The Cornea in Systemic Diseases

Some systemic diseases have important corneal manifestations. Examples are:

Disease	Corneal Manifestation
hypercalcemia and chronic *iridocyclitis*	calcium deposits (**band keratopathy**)
collagen diseases	corneal melting (ulceration)
syphilis	interstitial keratitis
cystinosis	corneal crystals
alkaptonuria	limbal and scleral pigmentation
Wilson's disease	Kayser-Fleischer ring
mucopolysaccharoidoses	corneal haze
leprosy	thick, beaded corneal nerves
Fabry's disease	vortex corneal dystrophy
amiodarone therapy } chloroquine therapy }	epithelial deposits similar to the vortex dystrophy of Fabry's disease
gout	uric acid crystals

Corneal Surgery

Corneal transplantation (penetrating keratoplasty) is the microsurgical placement of a healthy corneal "button" from a deceased donor into the diseased cornea of a patient. It is often done for *aphakic bullous keratopathy* (corneal clouding following cataract sur-

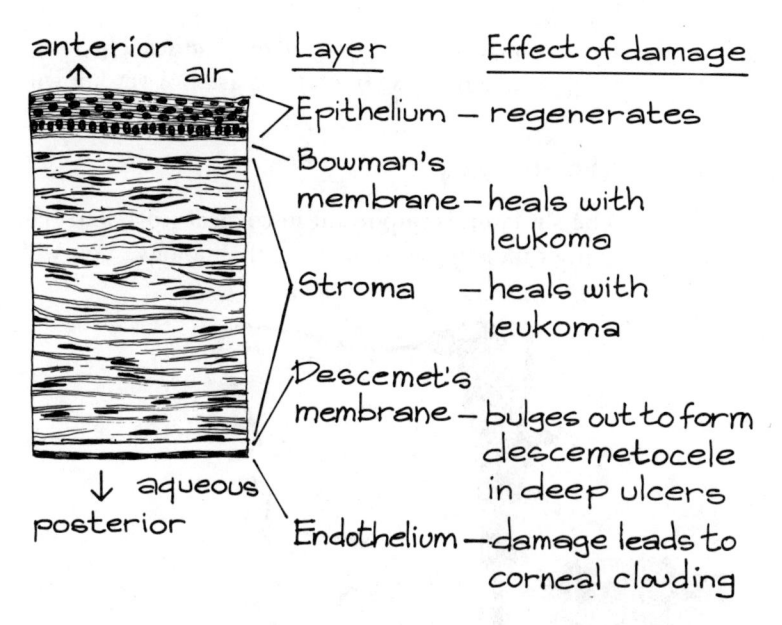

Layer	Effect of damage
Epithelium	regenerates
Bowman's membrane	heals with leukoma
Stroma	heals with leukoma
Descemet's membrane	bulges out to form descemetocele in deep ulcers
Endothelium	damage leads to corneal clouding

Corneal layers and effect of damage

gery). Other indications are *Fuchs' corneal dystrophy, keratoconus* and opacities due to trauma, inflammation, and congenital disease. Meticulous attention to patient selection, handling of donor material, surgical technique, and postoperative care are necessary to obtain a clear graft. **Lamellar keratoplasty** is a partial-thickness corneal transplant used in urgent cases of corneal perforation, corneal melting, superficial scars and defects, and complicated *pterygia*.

Refractive keratoplasty includes corneal operations such as **radial keratotomy** and **epikeratophakia**, which reshape the corneal surface to correct refractive errors, such as *myopia* and *astigmatism*. The long-term results of these operations are not yet known.

The Slit Lamp

The slit lamp is important in corneal work and has many other applications in opthalmology. You will

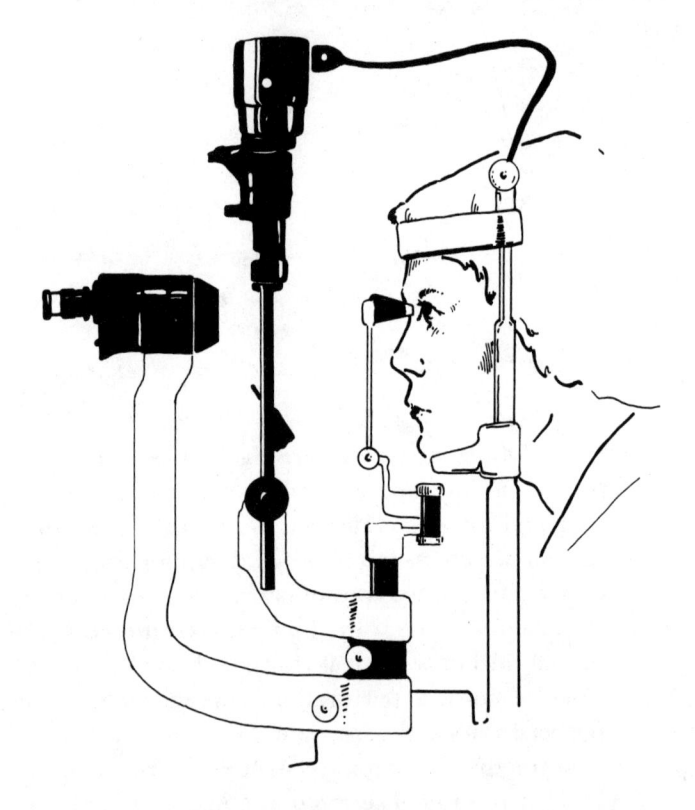

Slit lamp with applanation tonometer in place.

find that with a little practice it is easy to use. A slit of light creates an "optical section" so you can study the transparent cornea, anterior chamber, lens, and anterior vitreous as you would a cut tissue specimen. It also shows magnified details of the eyelids, conjunctiva, sclera, and iris.

Various procedures are done under the slit lamp, including removal of *corneal foreign bodies* (especially residual rust), suture removal, anterior chamber paracentesis, *laser iridotomy*, and *laser trabeculoplasty*.

Attachments make the slit lamp an even more versatile instrument:

Observation tube. This allows an observer to view along with the examiner.
Hruby lens. This gives a view of the posterior vitreous and central retina (optic disc, retinal vessels, macula).
Three-mirror contact lens. This permits a view of the central retina, anterior chamber angle (*gonioscopy*) and peripheral retina.
Applanation tonometer. This gives a direct reading of the intraocular pressure in mm Hg.
Pachometer. This measures the corneal thickness.
Camera. This is used for external photography, fundus photography, and *fluorescein angiography*.
Laser. The laser beam is directed into the eye by connecting the laser generating unit to a slit lamp mechanism.

14 The Retina and Vitreous

In patients complaining of poor vision, ophthalmoscopy often reveals retinal diseases with a characteristic appearance. Since in most areas the combined thickness of the choroid and retina is less than 0.5 mm, it is not surprising that most retinal diseases involve the choroid, and vice versa. Thus, *toxoplasmosis, histoplasmosis,* and *toxocariasis,* discussed here as diseases of the retina, are found in some texts under diseases of the choroid. Retinal vascular diseases are discussed in Chapter 7.

Age-Related Macular Degeneration

Age-related macular degeneration (AMD), also called **senile macular degeneration (SMD),** is the leading cause of acquired legal blindness in people over 60 years of age. In many older patients small yellow retinal bodies called **drusen** are seen in or near the macula. These excrescences are degenerative products of the retinal pigment epithelium. Macular drusen are usually asymptomatic but represent the beginning of macular degeneration. Periodic ophthalmoscopic examinations reveal gradual destruction of the macula.

Nonexudative ("dry," involutional or geographic) macular degeneration) is the most common form of AMD but only 10% of patients with legal blindness from AMD have this form of the disease.

Exudative ("wet or disciform") macular degeneration is less common but 90% of patients legally

Macular drusen

blind from AMD have the exudative type. Choroidal vessels in exudative AMD grow through breaks in Bruch's membrane to the subpigment epithelial and subretinal space. This is called **subretinal (or choroidal) neovascularization.** Subsequent hemorrhage and leakage from the abnormal vessels cause dete-

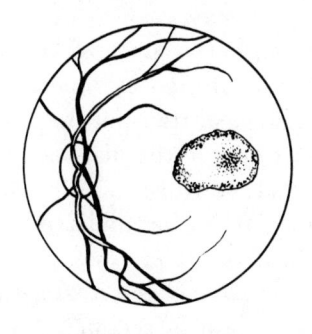

Disciform macular degeneration

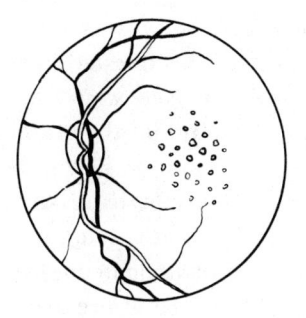

rioration of the overlying sensory retina. Subretinal neovascularization can be arrested in some patients by *argon* or *krypton laser photocoagulation* except when the vessels have grown under the center of the macula. Early treatment is more likely to be successful, so older patients with visual disturbances should be referred promptly for evaluation.

In patients with loss of vision in one eye, the chances of involvement of the second eye average 10% per year. The patient with advanced macular degeneration can be reassured that the disease is self-limited and that total blindness does not occur. Although reading small print and driving a car are impossible, peripheral vision remains, so that the patient can still see enough to get around. Large-print books and special reading aids often help these patients.

Toxoplasmosis

Toxoplasma gondii is a protozoan found in cats. Pregnant women infected by domestic cats or the ingestion of raw meat transmit the disease to their fetus. Three Cs help in the diagnosis of congenital toxoplasmosis: (1) *c*onvulsions; (2) *c*alcification (intracranial); and (3) *c*horioretinitis (more accurately: retinochoroiditis).

Childhood and adult ocular toxoplasmosis usually represent reactivation of retained *Toxoplasma* cysts from congenital infection. When the condition is acute, an ill-defined area of yellow-white retinochoroiditis is seen through hazy vitreous. Healed lesions

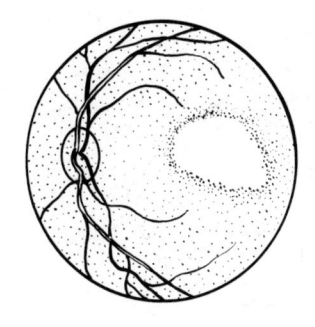

Acute toxoplasmosis
Area of retinochoroiditis
seen through hazy vitreous

are characteristic circumscribed areas of chorioretinal pigmentation and depigmentation. Macular involvement destroys central vision. Peripheral lesions may be asymptomatic. Hemagglutination or indirect fluorescent antibody tests help in diagnosis. Pyrimethamine, sulfadiazine, clindamycin, and steroids have been used in treatment.

Presumed Histoplasmic Chorioretinitis

Presumed histoplasmic chorioretinitis is more common where histoplasmosis is endemic, but although skin tests are usually positive, the *Histoplasma* fungus has never been isolated from a patient with the presumed ocular disease. A macular or circumpapillary

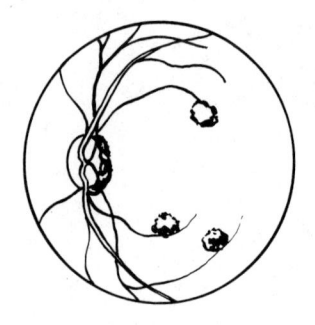

Old histoplasmosis peripapillary involvement and "histo spots"

scar is associated with hemorrhage and *subretinal neovascularization* with eventual destruction of the overlying retina. Pigmented and depigmented "histo spots" are scattered in the retina. Laser photocoagulation of the abnormal retinal vessels is of value in selected patients.

Toxocariasis

Toxocara canis is a nematode that grows in the gastrointestinal tract of dogs (especially puppies) and infects children who eat dirt. A single white granuloma the size of the optic disc or larger may be seen in or near the macula or elsewhere in the retina and can be mistaken for a *retinoblastoma*. The enzyme-linked immunosorbent assay (ELISA) test is a diagnostic aid. Other manifestations of ocular toxo-

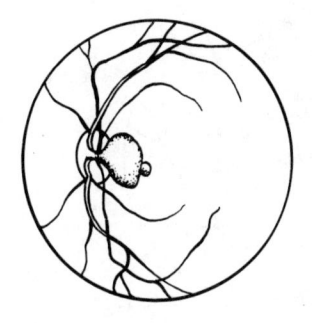

Toxocariasis
The worm has invaded the retina at the optic disc.

cariasis are endophthalmitis, cyclitis, or vitreoretinal bands. The nematode is occasionally observed moving beneath the retina. There is no uniformly effective treatment. Larval death may aggravate ocular inflammation.

Rhegmatogenous Retinal Detachment

Retinal detachment associated with retinal holes is known as rhegmatogenous retinal detachment. Degeneration of the vitreous and peripheral retina in old age, after cataract surgery or trauma, or in high myopia, may lead to one or more retinal holes (also called tears or breaks), usually caused by vitreous

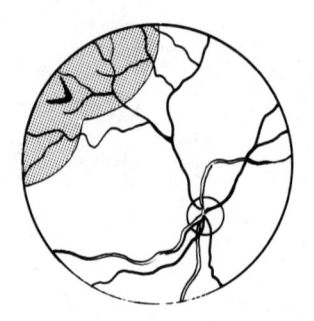

Retinal detachment

traction on the retina. Fluid vitreous leaks through the hole between the sensory retina and the pigment epithelium, so the retina becomes detached. Ophthalmoscopy reveals a partial or total elevation of the retina with an associated hole or holes. The resulting loss of peripheral vision is often described by the patient as a "shade" over the vision. If the macula is involved, central vision is obliterated. Surgery is usually successful, but vision may not return to 20/20. Without surgery the detachment becomes total and the eye eventually becomes sightless.

Nonrhegmatogenous Retinal Detachment

Two forms of retinal detachment occur without retinal holes: traction and exudative retinal detachment. **Traction retinal detachment** occurs in *retrolental fibroplasia, proliferative diabetic retinopathy,* and other diseases with vitreous traction on the retina. **Exudative (serous or secondary) retinal detachment** follows leakage of serum from choroidal or retinal vessels. This occurs with intraocular tumors, inflammations, or in chorioretinal degenerative diseases.

The Vitreous

The vitreous is involved in congenital abnormalities, injury, infection, degeneration, *proliferative diabetic retinopathy,* and retinal detachment.

Vitreous Detachment

The vitreous gel gradually contracts and liquefies with aging (**syneresis**). This produces detachment of the vitreous from the retina in most people by 65 years of age. Symptoms include flashes of light from vitreous traction on the retina and the sudden appearance of a cloud of vitreous floaters. The prognosis is good, since vision is not usually affected. The entire retina should be evaluated by careful *indirect ophthalmoscopy,* however, since retinal tears and retinal detachment are occasionally associated with vitreous detachment.

Vitrectomy

In vitrectomy operations a special small (usually 20 gauge) needle, with suction applied to a cutting tip, is inserted into the vitreous cavity of the eye. Most

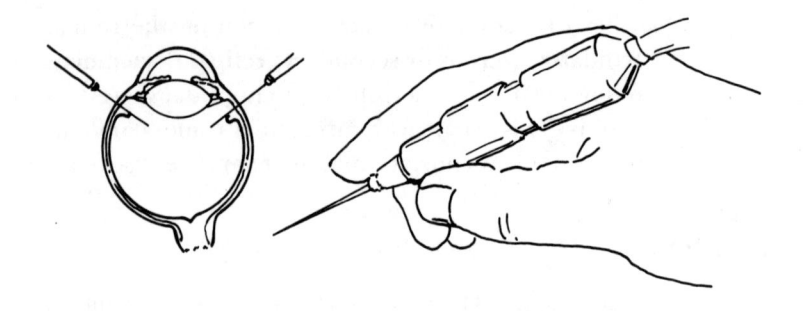

Vitrectomy

of the vitreous is removed by the suction and cutting action of the needle and is replaced with physiologic saline. The operation is performed with an operating microscope. The most common indications are *vitreous hemorrhage, ocular trauma,* and *traction retinal detachment* due to *proliferative diabetic retinopathy.* Vitrectomy is also employed in some patients with *endophthalmitis, retinal detachment,* and *intraocular foreign bodies.*

15 The Eye in Systemic Disease

Ocular abnormalities are important in many syndromes and systemic diseases. Examination of the eye often leads to a diagnosis. Some of these syndromes and diseases are listed alphabetically below. Others are described in the glossary.

Disease or Syndrome	Associated Abnormalities of the Eye
Abetalipoproteinemia (Bassen-Kornzweig syndrome)	Night blindness; pigmentary retinopathy
Alport syndrome (hereditary nephritis and deafness)	Anterior lenticonus
Ataxia telangiectasia (Louis-Bar syndrome—cerebellar ataxia and sinopulmonary infection)	Conjunctival telangiectasia; oculomotor apraxia
Atopic dermatitis	Keratoconus; cataract; vernal conjunctivitis; herpes keratitis
Beri-beri (vitamin B deficiency; Wernicke's encephalopathy)	Central scotoma; diplopia, nystagmus
Cogan syndrome	Interstitial keratitis with deafness and vertigo
Crohn's disease	Episcleritis; uveitis
Cystinosis	Cystine crystals in cornea
Cytomegalovirus inclusion disease	Retinitis, uveitis

Disease or Syndrome	Associated Abnormalities of the Eye
Dermatomyositis	Heliotrope discoloration of eyelids
Ehlers-Danlos syndrome (hyperelastic skin; loose joints)	Epicanthal folds; angioid streaks in retina; retinal hemorrhage; ptosis; eversion of upper eyelid
Fabry syndrome (skin angiectases due to ceramide trihexoside accumulation)	Vortex corneal dystrophy
Fractures of long bones	Purtscher's retinopathy: bilateral multiple cotton-wool spots due to fat emboli
Galactosemia	Infantile cataract
Homocystinuria	Dislocated lens
Hyperlipoproteinemia	Xanthelasma; lipemia retinalis
Hypoparathyroidism	Cataract
Incontinentia pigmenti (Bloch-Sulzberger syndrome: pigmented skin lesions, eosinophilia, dental anomalies, alopecia)	Strabismus; cataract; optic atrophy; blue sclera; uveitis; retinal dysplasia
Laurence-Moon-Biedl syndrome (obesity; mental retardation; polydactyly; hypogonadism)	Retinitis pigmentosa

Disease or Syndrome	Associated Abnormalities of the Eye
Leprosy	Scleritis; keratitis; uveitis; retinitis; neuropathy of cranial nerves 5 and 7
Leukemia	Retinal hemorrhage; Roth spots; proptosis
Lupus erythematosus	Cotton-wool retinal exudates; optic neuritis
Mandibulofacial dysostosis (Franceschetti syndrome; Treacher-Collins syndrome)	Antimongoloid palpebral fissures; eyelid colobomas; sagging of lower eyelids; absence of cilia and lacrimal puncta
Möbius syndrome	Congenital unilateral or bilateral paralysis of cranial nerves 6 and 7
Multiple myeloma	Dilated retinal veins; retinal vein occlusion
Onchocerciasis (river blindness)	Conjunctivitis; interstitial keratitis. After treatment: chemosis and lid edema (Manzotti reaction)
Osteogenesis imperfecta (van der Hoeve syndrome; brittle bones; blue sclera; deafness)	Blue sclera; megalocornea; keratoconus; cataract; embryotoxon
Pemphigoid	Conjunctival shrinkage; symblepharon; episcleritis; uveitis

Disease or Syndrome	Associated Abnormalities of the Eye
Polyarteritis nodosa	Retinal vasculitis; marginal corneal ulcer
Polycythemia	Engorged conjunctival and retinal vessels; retinal vein occlusion
Pseudoxanthoma elasticum (Grönblad-Strandberg syndrome: thick yellow skin, arterial degeneration and hemorrhage)	Angioid streaks in retina
Rothmund-Thompson syndrome (ectodermal dysplasia)	Cataract
Scleroderma	Sjögren syndrome
Sickle cell disease	Proliferative vascular retinopathy
Still's disease	Band keratopathy; cataract
Syphilis	Argyll Robertson pupil; interstitial keratitis; chorioretinitis
Tay-Sachs disease (amaurotic family idiocy)	Cherry-red spot in macula; retinal degeneration
Vitamin A deficiency	Bitot's spot; keratomalacia; night blindness; xerophthalmia
Waldenstrom's macroglobulinemia	Dilated retinal veins; retinal vein occlusion

Disease or Syndrome	Associated Abnormalities of the Eye
Wilson's disease (hepatolenticular degeneration)	Kayser-Fleischer corneal ring; sunflower cataract
Wyburn-Mason syndrome	Racemose hemangioma of retina; midbrain hemangioma
Xeroderma pigmentosum	Basal and squamous carcinoma of eyelids

16 Special Diagnostic Studies

Fluorescein Angiography

In fluorescein angiography fluorescein is injected into the antecubital vein. Rapid-sequence photography records ocular blood flow, vascular leaks, other vascular abnormalities, and defects in the retinal pigment epithelium. *Diabetic retinopathy, intraocular tumors, retinal vein occlusion, macular degeneration,* and many other diseases are studied with this technique.

Electroretinogram

The electroretinogram (ERG) records small voltage changes that occur when light strikes the retina. It is a response of the entire retina and may be normal even if part of the retina is damaged. The ERG is valuable in detecting retinal function in retinal detachment when the ocular media are opaque. It is abnormal in retinitis pigmentosa. The ERG is not affected in glaucoma except in its most advanced stage.

Electro-oculogram

The electro-oculogram (EOG) utilizes the minute current generated by eye movements. An abnormal EOG reflects disease of the retinal pigment epithelium. For example, the EOG is important in the diagnosis of **Best's vitelliform degeneration.** Early in this hereditary disease there is an egg-yolk appearance to the macula. Characteristically the EOG is abnormal and the ERG is normal.

Photopic ERG

EOG

VEP

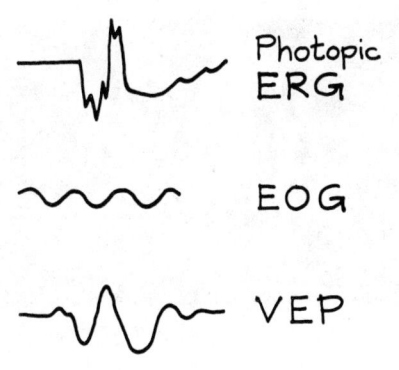

Visual Evoked Potential

The visual evoked potential (VEP) is recorded from the occipital lobe with equipment similar to that used in the EEG. Reduction in vision from macular and optic nerve disease can be quantitated in children and adults.

Computed Tomography

The computed tomography (CT) scan permits excellent radiologic visualization of ocular and orbital tumors and other pathologic changes in the eye and orbit. The appearance of the CT scan often suggests a pathologic diagnosis.

Magnetic Resonance Imaging

MR imaging is a noninvasive technique that shows details of the eye and orbit like the CT scan without

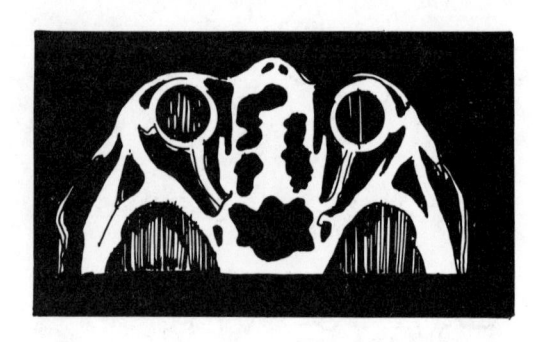

Orbital CT scan

X-radiation. There is good soft-tissue contrast. Bone shows up as empty space with MR imaging but soft-tissue tumors invading bone are demonstrated.

Ultrasound

Ultrasound is useful when it is impossible to see into the eye and like the CT scan and MR imaging may

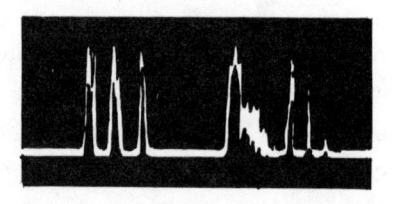

A-scan ultrasonogram

B-scan ultrasonogram

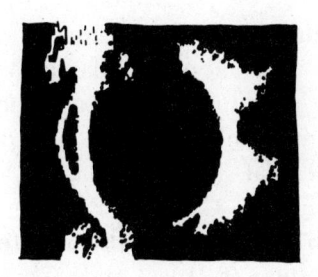

suggest a specific diagnosis. The **A scan ultrasonogram** gives an idea of the location and density of ocular and orbital tumors and of the presence of retinal detachment. It is also used to measure the length of the eye to help determine the power of intraocular lens implants. The **B scan ultrasonogram** suggests the shape and location of ocular orbital tumors.

Ultrasound is less expensive than the CT scan and MR imaging. Like MR imaging it involves no radiation exposure. The CT scan or MR imaging provide the most accurate visualization, but ultrasound studies should also be done in all orbital and ocular tumors.

17 Lasers in Ophthalmology

The ophthalmic laser is a source of amplified coherent light mounted on a slit lamp. When directed into the eye, it produces **photocoagulation** burns that are accurate in number, location, size, duration, and intensity. Several kinds of lasers are used in ophthalmology.

The argon laser is commonly used for **panretinal photocoagulation (PRP)** in *proliferative diabetic retinopathy*. Over a thousand burns are scattered throughout the retina. This stops the growth of abnormal vessels into the vitreous which otherwise can cause blindness from *vitreous hemorrhage* or *traction retinal detachment* (See Chapter 7).

Subretinal neovascularization in *macular degeneration* and *ocular histoplasmosis* is also treated with the argon laser (see Chapter 14).

Iris neovascularization (*rubeosis iridis*) is seen in diabetics and, in some patients, after *central retinal vein occlusion*. Secondary glaucoma occurs when these abnormal vessels involve the *anterior chamber angle*. Like retinal neovascularization, abnormal iris vessels can be obliterated indirectly with argon laser PRP.

Open-angle glaucoma is often treated by argon laser *trabeculoplasty*. A *gonioscopic* lens is placed on the cornea to direct the laser into the *anterior chamber angle*. The laser burns alter the *trabecular meshwork* so that aqueous drainage is improved.

The krypton laser is used for photocoagulation close to the fovea since it is less likely to damage central nerve fibers. It is also useful when the ocular media are cloudy from hemorrhage or cataract.

The **neodymium-YAG laser** creates a short-pulsed "microexplosion" that accurately disrupts the posterior lens capsule, which may become opaque after extracapsular cataract surgery. The laser creates a hole in the opaque membrane, which restores clear vision.

The **carbon dioxide laser** cuts by vaporizing tissue water. It is used for various oculoplastic procedures. Unlike other ophthalmic lasers, the laser beam comes from a handle held by the surgeon.

Lasers are a useful adjunct in ophthalmology. Some patients, however, because of media publicity, believe lasers can restore vision in any eye disease. Careful explanation is necessary, since ophthalmic lasers are used only in special circumstances.

18 Common Misunderstandings About the Eye

1. **Incorrect:** Television, dim lights, incorrect glasses, reading too close, or overuse of the eyes damages the eyes.
   Correct: Eye fatigue or *asthenopia* is the only result.
2. **Incorrect:** Cataracts have to be mature for surgery.
   Correct: Cataracts can be removed at any stage.
3. **Incorrect:** Contact lens wear can cure myopia.
   Correct: Myopia returns after contact lenses are discontinued.
4. **Incorrect:** Farsighted (hyperopic) people see better at a distance.
   Correct: They see the same or worse than an emmetrope.
5. **Incorrect:** Eyewashes are good for the eye.
   Correct: Eyewashes are not necessary. Frequent use can cause eye irritation.
6. **Incorrect:** Old people who read without glasses have exceptionally healthy eyes.
   Correct: They have either common myopia or acquired myopia from cataract.
7. **Incorrect:** The "colored" part of the eye is on the surface of the eye.
   Correct: The pigmented iris is inside the eye, covered by the transparent cornea.
8. **Incorrect:** The eye is often removed for eye surgery.

Common Misunderstandings About the Eye

  Correct: This is never done. Removal of the eye causes blindness.
9. **Incorrect:** Eye pain is a common sign of glaucoma.
  Correct: Pain in the eye is only occasionally due to acute glaucoma. Most glaucoma patients have no pain.
10. **Incorrect:** Trouble learning to read is usually due to eye disease or need for glasses.
  Correct: Reading difficulty is more often due to low intelligence, emotional problems, or *dyslexia*.
11. **Incorrect:** Eye exercises improve vision and promote healthy eyes.
  Correct: Eye exercises do not correct refractive errors and are not necessary for eye health.

Glossary

Adie's pupil Physiologic opposite of *Horner syndrome*. Paralysis of parasympathetic nerves leads to a dilated pupil that responds slowly to light. It is usually seen in females with diminished tendon reflexes and has a good prognosis.

Adnexa Appendages, as in ocular adnexa; the eyelids, lacrimal apparatus, and other appendages of the eye.

Amaurosis Blindness, especially from systemic cause outside the eye—for example, toxic amaurosis from methyl alcohol poisoning.

Amaurosis fugax Transient monocular blindness. Causes are carotid atherosclerosis, cerebrovascular insufficiency, papilledema, migraine, or any condition associated with decreased arterial perfusion of the visual system.

Amblyopia Dimness of vision with no detectable lesion of the eye.

Angioid streaks Irregular pigmented streaks radiating from the optic disc in the retina; associated with pseudoxanthoma elasticum, sickle cell disease, Paget's disease, and Ehlers-Danlos syndrome.

Anisocoria Unequal pupil size. The pupils are slightly unequal in about 20% of normal individuals. If the inequality is significant, the physician must determine whether the smaller or larger pupil is abnormal.

Anterior chamber angle Angle where the posterior cornea meets the anterior iris. Narrowing of this angle may block the normal drainage of aqueous and lead to *acute narrow-angle glaucoma*.

Anterior chamber cleavage syndrome Mesenchymal dysgenesis of the anterior segment. This syndrome consists of thinning and opacities of the central posterior cornea, adhesions of the iris to the cornea, lens opacities, and abnormalities of the anterior chamber angle. Related are Rieger syndrome, Peters' anomaly, and Axenfeld syndrome.

Anterior segment Cornea, anterior chamber, iris, pupil, and lens.

Aphakia Absence of lens, as after cataract surgery.

Aphakic bullous keratopathy Cloudy cornea from damage to the corneal endothelium at the time of cataract surgery.

Arcus senilis Bilateral lipid infiltration of the cornea in a circular zone near the limbus, frequent in older individuals. In middle-aged persons with arcus senilis, blood lipids are often elevated.

Argyll Robertson pupil Small pupil that does not respond to light; seen in CNS lues. The initials help in remembering the characteristic signs: APR, Accommodation Reflex Present; and backwards, PRA, Pupillary Reflex Absent.

Glossary

Asteroid hyalosis Condition in which numerous small yellow spheres containing calcium soaps are suspended in the vitreous. Vision remains good.

Asthenopia Eyestrain.

Behçet syndrome Severe uveitis with hypopyon associated with ulcers of mouth and genitalia.

Bell's phenomenon Normal upward movement of the eyes when the eyelids are squeezed shut.

Berlin's edema Edema of retina after trauma.

Bitot spot Bulbar conjunctival plaques in the interpalpebral fissure caused by vitamin A deficiency.

Blepharochalasis Baggy eyelids. More specifically, an allergic eyelid swelling of children with secondary baggy eyelid skin.

blepharophimosis Congenital syndrome with blepharoptosis, narrow palpebral apertures, telecanthus, and epicanthus.

Blepharospasm Involuntary spastic closure of eyelids. Severe cases are treated with partial section of the facial nerve, removal of the orbicularis oculi muscles, or injection of botulinum toxin into the eyelids.

Blind spot Normal defect in the visual field where the optic nerve enters the eye.

Brown syndrome Restriction of action of the superior oblique muscle usually due to abnormalities of its tendon or tendon sheath.

Bulbar   Refers to the eyeball.

Bullous keratopathy   Edematous corneal blebs in advanced glaucoma, *Fuchs' dystrophy*, and *aphakic bullous keratopathy*, caused by decompensated, damaged corneal endothelium.

Buphthalmos   Enlargement of the eye in congenital glaucoma. The abnormal cornea has a diameter greater than 11 mm.

Canal of Schlemm   Canal encircling the eye close to the *trabecular meshwork*. Aqueous drains through the trabecular meshwork into the canal of Schlemm and then into veins in the sclera.

Canthus   Angle at either end of the opening between the eyelids.

Carotid-cavernous fistula   Rupture of the carotid artery in the cavernous sinus as a result of head injury or atherosclerosis. Pulsating exophthalmos, ocular bruit, headache, *chemosis*, dilated conjunctival vessels, and decreased vision occur on the involved side. Treatment includes intracranial or extracranial carotid artery ligation or intravascular introduction of a balloon or embolic material.

Central serous chorioretinopathy   Idiopathic serous detachment of the retinal pigment epithelium under the fovea producing distorted and blurred vision (*metamorphopsia*). The condition usually improves in several months but may recur, causing permanent loss of vision.

Chemosis Edema of the conjunctiva seen in inflammation from any cause.

Chlamydia (formerly called TRIC viruses). Obligate intracellular parasites that cause trachoma, adult and neonatal *inclusion conjunctivitis*, and lymphogranuloma venereum.

Choroidal detachment Elevation of the choroid and attached retina due to effusion of serous fluid between the choroid and the sclera. The characteristic smooth elevation seen by ophthalmoscopy differentiates the condition from a retinal detachment. It is associated with *hypotony* and may follow ocular surgery, trauma, and various eye diseases.

Choroideremia Sex-linked recessive disease that causes night blindness in males in the first decade of life. Atrophy of the choroid and retina begins at the periphery and eventually produces severe visual disability.

Circinate retinopathy Condition characterized by yellow exudates in a circular pattern around the macula.

Coloboma Congenital absence of part of the eyelid, iris, choroid, or retina.

Corectopia Displacement of the pupil from its normal central position.

Corneal limbus Periphery of the cornea where it joins the sclera.

Crouzon syndrome Congenital froglike facies with hypertelorism.

Circumpapillary Around the optic disc.

Cylinder Cylindrical lens used to correct astigmatism. (*Cf. sphere.*)

Cystoid macular edema (CME) Edema of the macula after cataract surgery. The condition can produce significant loss of vision, which may gradually improve or be permanent. It is more common after intracapsular cataract extraction and with dipivefrin treatment of aphakic glaucoma.

Demodex follicularum Mite often present in eyelash follicles; in large numbers, a cause of blepharitis.

Dislocated lens Condition seen in trauma, syphilis, and various congenital diseases such as Marfan syndrome and homocystinuria.

Distichiasis Condition in which congenital abnormal eyelashes grow from the meibomian orifices and irritate the cornea.

Drusen (1) Degenerative yellow spots usually in the region of the macula. (2) Nodular bodies close to the optic disc that may be confused with papilledema.

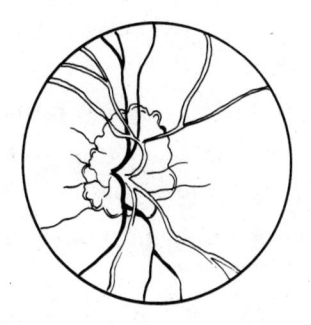

Drusen of the optic disc

Duane syndrome Condition in which attempted adduction of the eye results in narrowing of the lid fissure and enophthalmos.

Dyslexia Inability to read due to a congenital CNS defect. Parents should be skeptical about long, costly treatment programs.

Ectropion Condition in which the lower eyelid sags or is turned out. Tearing and irritation oc-

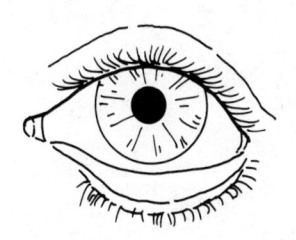

Ectropion

cur from exposure of the eye. Uncommon in the upper eyelid.

Embryotoxon Ringlike opacity of the cornea.

Emmetrope Person who has no refractive error and thus does not need glasses.

Endophthalmitis Inflammation of all the internal structures of the eye.

Endothelium In the cornea, the innermost layer. Any damage from injury, surgery, or disease will result in corneal clouding.

Enophthalmos Condition in which the eye retracts into the orbit. The opposite of *exophthalmos* or *proptosis*.

Entropion Condition in which the upper or lower eyelid turns in. *Trichiasis* is usually associated.

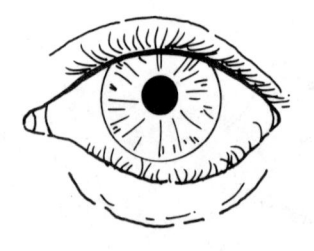

Entropion

Enucleation Surgical removal of the eyeball (muscles, fat, lids, and conjunctiva are preserved).

Epicanthus Fold over the medial canthus. Normal in infants.

Epiphora Tearing. Bilateral epiphora can be caused by any eye irritation. In unilateral epiphora suspect mechanical obstruction.

Essential iris atrophy Rare entity consisting of progressive loss of iris stroma, pupil distortion, and severe glaucoma.

Evisceration Surgical removal of the contents of the eye; the scleral shell remains, along with all the other structures of the orbit.

Exenteration With reference to the eye, removal of the entire contents of the orbit: eye, muscles, eyelids, fat. Used for advanced cancer.

Fluorescein Fluorescent dye used in determining the fit of contact lenses, in the detection of corneal damage, and, injected intravenously, in the study of diseases of the choroid and retina (*fluorescein angiogram*).

Fluorescein strip Fluorescein-impregnated paper in individual sterile package.

Fuchs' dystrophy Degeneration of the corneal endothelium that leads to abnormal corneal hydration and loss of corneal transparency.

Dystrophy   Trachomatous pannus   Leukoma

Interstitial keratitis   Pterygium   Arcus Senilis

Some chronic corneal abnormalities

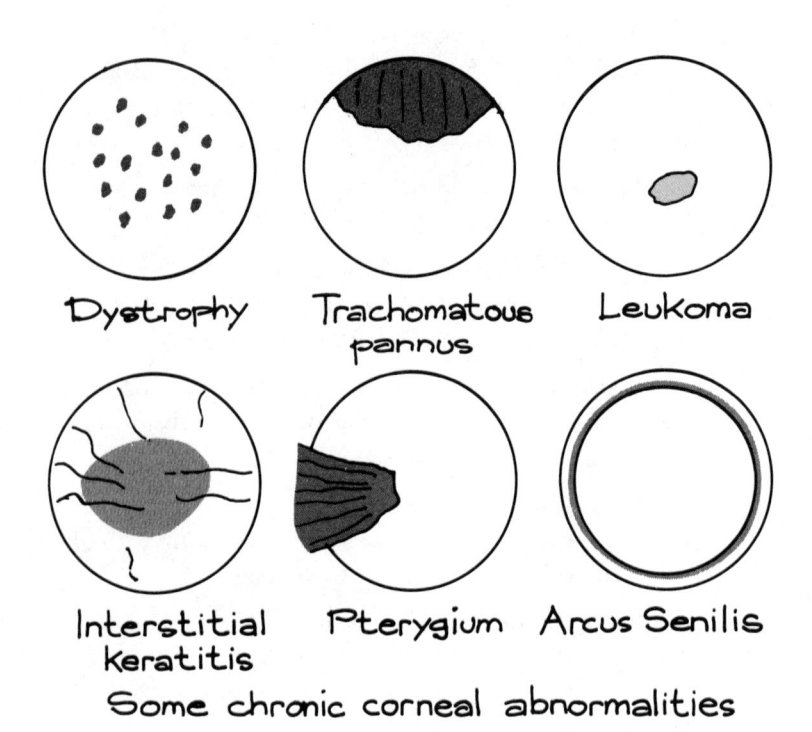

Fundus   Interior of a hollow organ such as the eye.

Globe   Eyeball.

Goldenhar syndrome   Oculo-auricular vertebral dysplasia. Characterized by epibulbar dermoids, accessory auricular appendages, and vertebral abnormalities.

Goldman-Favre disease   Congenital vitreoretinal degeneration with severe loss of vision from retinoschisis, atypical retinitis pigmentosa, and cataract.

Gonioscopy Examination of the anterior chamber angle of the eye. A special corneal contact (gonioscopic) lens is used.

Gyrate atrophy Progressive patchy atrophy of the choroid and retina similar to *choroideremia* in appearance and symptomatology. Unlike choroideremia, it is inherited as a recessive trait.

Hamartoma Benign overgrowth of cells and tissues.

Heterochromia of the iris Condition in which the iris color differs in the two eyes. It occurs as a congenital anomaly, with congenital Horner syndrome, and with heterochromic iritis.

Horton syndrome Cluster headaches. Periodic unilateral headache with pain, redness, and tearing of the eye.

Hypertelorism Abnormally increased distance between the orbits as determined by X-ray measurement (*cf. telecanthus*).

Hypotony Decreased intraocular pressure. Causes are fistula secondary to trauma or surgery, phthisis bulbi, choroidal detachment, glaucoma medications, hyperosmotic agents, and hyposecretion of the ciliary body from any cause.

Interstitial keratitis Cloudy cornea with stromal vascularization. Congenital lues is the most common cause.

Iridectomy Surgical excision of part of the iris.

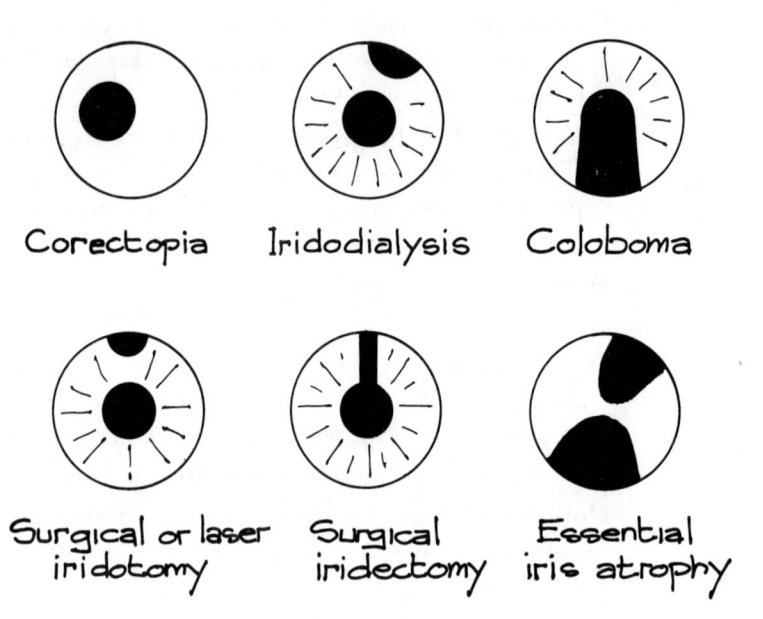

Corectopia   Iridodialysis   Coloboma

Surgical or laser iridotomy   Surgical iridectomy   Essential iris atrophy

Some iris abnormalities

Iridodialysis Separation of the iris from its attachment (often traumatic).

Iridodonesis Tremulous iris in aphakia or dislocated lens.

Iridotomy Creation of a small opening in the base of the iris. Done for the treatment of narrow-angle glaucoma or prophylactically, at the time of cataract surgery, to facilitate the flow of aqueous from the posterior to the anterior chamber.

Juvenile retinoschisis Sex-linked congenital disease with splitting of the retina peripherally and in the macular area.

Kayser-Fleischer ring Pigmented corneal ring in Wilson's disease.

Keratitis Any inflammation of the cornea from trauma or disease.

Keratoconjunctivitis sicca (KCS) Dry eyes from tear deficiency; a common cause of irritative conjunctivitis in middle-aged women. (See *Sjögren syndrome.*)

Keratoconus Conical protrusion of the central part of the cornea. Contact lenses improve vision in mild cases. A corneal transplant is required in severe cases.

Keratoprosthesis Plastic corneal implant used in severe corneal disease when a conventional corneal transplant is impossible.

Kuhnt-Junius disease *Disciform macular degeneration.*

Lagophthalmos Delayed or incomplete eyelid closure, as from seventh nerve paralysis.

Lamellar With reference to the cornea, partial thickness, as in lamellar corneal transplant.

Lattice degeneration of the cornea *Corneal dystrophy* with a characteristic pattern of amyloid deposition in the corneal stroma.

Lattice degeneration of the retina Peripheral retinal degeneration associated with retinal detachment.

Leber's hereditary optic atrophy Recessive sex-linked optic atrophy affecting males in their early 20s. Loss of central vision in one eye is followed by involvement of the other eye. Peripheral vision is retained.

Leukocoria White pupil from cataract, congenital abnormality, or tumor.

Leukoma White opacity of the cornea.

Marcus Gunn jaw-winking phenomenon Movement of a ptotic eyelid up and down when chewing.

Melanosis oculi Abnormal pigmentation of the eye or ocular adnexa.

Microphthalmos Developmental defect in which the eyeball is abnormally small.

Mohs fresh-tissue surgery Removal of skin cancer under local anesthetic in the dermatologist's office. Repeated excisions are done until frozen microscopic sections show that all cancerous tissue has been removed.

Mucopolysaccharidoses Genetic defects of mucopolysaccharide metabolism with skeletal changes, mental retardation, visceral involvement, corneal clouding, and urinary secretion of mucopolysaccharides.

Myasthenia gravis Disorder of neuromuscular function. Blepharoptosis and diplopia are often the first signs. Weakness of facial and other muscles follows. Intravenous edrophonium for diagnosis temporarily relieves the ptosis and ocular muscle weakness.

Myelinated (medullated) nerve fibers Harmless opaque white patch with feathery edges extending from the optic disc in about 0.5% of normal eyes; occasionally associated with myopia strabismus and *amblyopia*.

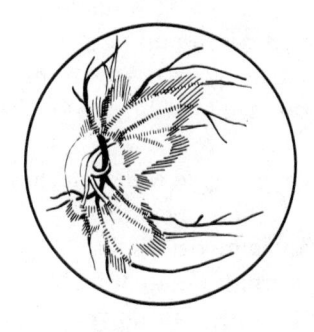

Myelinated nerve fibers

Myotonic dystrophy Hereditary muscle wasting associated with cataracts, testicular atrophy, and baldness.

Ocularist Professional whose full-time occupation is the fabrication of artificial eyes and related prostheses.

Oculist Old term for ophthalmologist.

Oculus, oculi [*Latin*] Eye.

Ophthalmo- [*Greek*] Combining form denoting relationship to the eye.

Ophthalmologist Physician with an M.D. degree who has had three years postgraduate training in diseases and surgery of the eye.

Ophthalmoplegia Paralysis of the extraocular muscles (EOM) or pupil.
  Total: EOM paralysis with a dilated pupil. The eye is deviated down and out; the upper eyelid is ptotic. Unruptured aneurysm of the internal carotid artery is the most common cause.
  External: Same as above with a normal pupil. Diabetes is a common cause.
  Internal: Paralytic mydriasis.
  Progressive external: Gradual inability to move the eyes with ptosis, but normal pupil reactions. When associated with *retinitis pigmentosa,* deafness, heart block, and peripheral neuropathy it is called **ophthalmoplegia plus** or the Kearns-Sayre syndrome.

Ophthalmoscope, binocular indirect Ophthalmoscope mounted on a headband and used with a condensing lens held close to the patient's eye. The retinal image is inverted and smaller than that obtained with the direct ophthalmoscope, but is three-dimensional. An experienced exam-

Glossary

iner can visualize the entire retina with this instrument.

Ophthalmoscope, direct Hand-held ophthalmoscope that gives an upright image of the retina magnified 15 times.

Optic atrophy Atrophy of the optic disc resulting from degeneration of the fibers of the optic nerve and optic tract. A flat, white optic disc seen on ophthalmoscopy indicates a functionless optic nerve from end stage vascular occlusion, papilledema, optic neuritis, trauma, tumors, glaucoma, toxicity, or degenerative disease.

Optician One who fits glasses or contact lenses on the prescription of an ophthalmologist or optometrist.

Optokinetic drum Drum with alternating black and white stripes on its surface, mounted on a handle so it can be rotated. Nystagmus normally occurs when a patient looks at the rotating drum (*optokinetic nystagmus*).

Optometrist (O.D.) A specialist in examination and treatment of the eye with glasses, contact lenses, and visual training. Optometrists do not perform surgery. Laws have been passed in some states allowing optometrists to use some drugs.

Orbital apex syndrome (Rollet syndrome) An extension of the *sphenoidal fissure syndrome,* with the addition of visual loss, papilledema, and optic atrophy due to optic nerve involvement.

Osteopath (D.O.) Doctor of osteopathy. Some osteopathic physicians specialize in ophthalmology.

Panophthalmitis Inflammation of all the structures of the eye.

Papillary In ophthalmology, refers to optic disc (optic papilla).

Perimeter An arc-shaped or bowl-shaped instrument for measuring the peripheral field of vision.

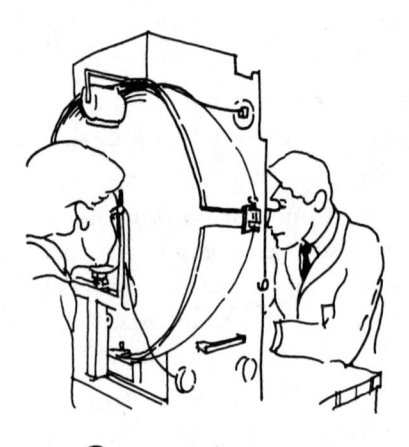

Perimetry

Peripapillary Around the optic disc.

Phacomatoses Classically the following four syndromes are called phacomatoses. Related syndromes are called **disseminated hamartomas**, the preferred term for the entire group. Dominant hereditary transmission is characteristic.

Von Hippel-Landau disease Angiomatosis of the retina; hemangioblastoma of the cerebellum, medulla, and spinal cord; and cysts of the kidney and pancreas.

Tuberous sclerosis (Bourneville disease) Epilepsy, mental deficiency, fibrous angiomas of the skin, and mulberry tumors of the retina.

Neurofibromatosis (Von Recklinghausen disease) Multiple cutaneous neurofibromas occur with cafe-au-lait spots of the skin and neurogenic tumors of the eyelids, orbit, retina, and central nervous system. Optic nerve glioma, meningioma, and acoustic neuroma (cerebellopontine angle tumor) are associated.

Sturge-Weber syndrome Portwine nevus of the area of facial skin supplied by the trigeminal nerve, choroidal angioma, and glaucoma.

Phthisis bulbi Shrunken blind eye.

Pinguecula Thickened, raised conjunctival tissue near the sclerocorneal junction in the 3 or 9 o'clock position.

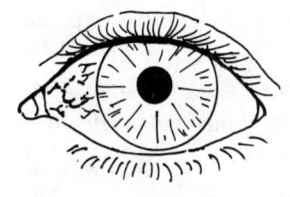

Pinguecula

Posterior chamber Small space posterior to the iris. Aqueous secreted by the ciliary body into the posterior chamber passes through the pupil into the *anterior chamber*.

Posterior pole Macula and fovea of the retina. Destruction of the macula or fovea by disease or injury results in loss of central vision.

Pseudoptosis Ptosis with a normal upper eyelid. One cause is hypotropia (downward deviation of the eye). When the hypotropic eye is forced to fixate by covering the normal eye, the ptosis disappears. Pseudoptosis occurs when the eyelid lacks support after enucleation or with a shrunken (phthisical) eye. Tumors and inflammatory disease of the eyelids or orbit often produce pseudoptosis.

Pseudostrabismus Many babies referred to an ophthalmologist for strabismus have pseudostrabismus, since the normal infant epicanthal fold often makes the eye look crossed. Refer if in doubt, since patching in true strabismus will prevent *amblyopia ex anopsia*.

Pterygium Wedge of conjunctival scarlike tissue growing into the cornea from the nasal side from ultraviolet light or dust exposure. Surgery is indicated for progressive growth. Recurrence after surgery is common. Ultraviolet light–blocking sunglasses should be worn.

Raeder syndrome Pain in the eye and head with Horner syndrome.

Refsum syndrome Atypical retinitis pigmentosa, night blindness, polyneuritis, ataxia, weakness, increased CSF protein, and abnormal phytanic acid metabolism.

Reiter syndrome Uveitis or conjunctivitis with urethritis and arthritis.

Retinitis pigmentosa (RP) Hereditary, bilateral degeneration of the retina with multiple areas of "bone corpuscle" pigment degeneration leads to progressive night blindness, contraction of the visual fields, and loss of vision. It can be associated with other congenital abnormalities such as *ophthalmoplegia* polyneuritis, deafness, and heart block. (See *Refsum syndrome, Kearns-Sayre syndrome,* and *progressive external ophthalmoplegia.*)

Retinoschisis Splitting of the retina in two layers from a hereditary dystrophy or a senile degeneration.

Retrolental fibroplasia (RLF) (Also called **retinitis of prematurity (ROP)** Absolute or relative oxygen excess leading to neovascularization and fibrosis of the peripheral retina in infants with low birth weight. Traction on the macula and pseudostrabismus occur in mild cases, and *traction detachment of the retina* and blindness in severe cases.

Roth spots Retinal hemorrhages with a white center made up of leukocytes or fibrin. They were once thought to be specific for subacute bacterial endocarditis but can occur with retinal

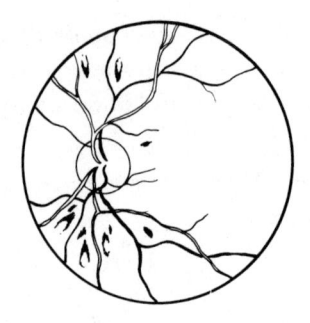

Roth spots in pernicious anemia

hemorrhages from leukemia or pernicious anemia.

Rubeosis iridis New vessels in the iris associated with diabetes, central retinal vein occlusion, and carotid occlusive disease. If the anterior chamber angle is involved, intractable secondary glaucoma results.

Schematic (or reduced) eye Diagram of the eye to show its optics in simplified form.

Schirmer test Strips of filter paper placed in the conjunctival sac should wet 10–15 mm in five minutes. If significantly less, tear deficiency exists, as in *Sjögren syndrome* and other dry eye conditions.

Scotoma Blind or partially blind area in the visual field.

Sjögren syndrome *Keratoconjunctivitis sicca,* rheumatoid arthritis, and dry mouth.

Speed reading Reading speed can be improved with training and practice. This is effective in fiction and newspaper text, but less so for scientific and technical material.

Sphenoidal fissure syndrome Inflammation or tumor in the region of the sphenoid fissure causes pain, proptosis, ocular palsies, and diplopia due to involvement of cranial nerves passing through sphenoidal (superior orbital) fissure (cranial nerves 3, 4, and 6).

Sphere Lens used to correct hyperopia (plus sphere) or myopia (minus sphere) (*cf. cylinder*).

Staphyloma Bulging of thin sclera secondary to *scleritis*.

Stargardt disease Hereditary retinal dystrophy that occurs about age 8–14 and first causes loss of central vision. Later, degenerative changes develop in the macula.

Symblepharon Adhesion between the bulbar and palpebral conjunctiva.

Sympathetic ophthalmia Granulomatous inflammation of the uveal tract of the uninjured (sympathizing) eye that occurs weeks, months, or years after a wound of the uveal tract of the injured (exciting) eye. Bilateral granulomatous panuveitis and blindness may result. Cases today are rare and the prognosis is better with steroid and antimetabolite therapy.

Synchysis scintilans Condition in which numerous cholesterol crystals settle in fluid vitreous and fly around the vitreous cavity when the eye moves. They are nonprogressive and vision remains good.

Tolosa-Hunt syndrome Painful ophthalmoplegia attributed to inflammation in the cavernous sinus or sphenoidal fissure.

Tangent screen Large square of black cloth, used with test objects to map the central field of vision.

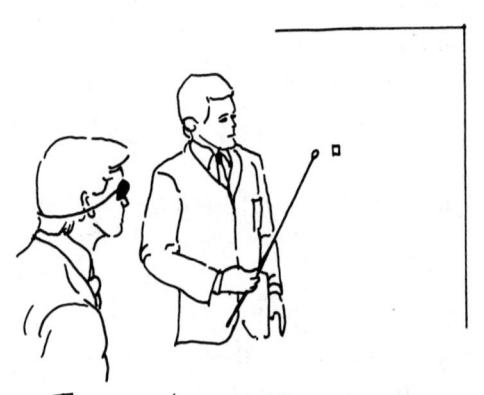

Tangent screen examination

Tarsorrhaphy Operation in which the eyelids are partially or completely sewn shut to protect the cornea.

Tarsus Framework of connective tissue which gives shape and support to the eyelids.

Telecanthus Increased distance between the medial canthi easily determined by external measurement (*cf. hypertelorism*).

Glossary

Tonography Recording of changes in intraocular pressure produced by the constant application of a known weight on the globe of the eye in evaluation of glaucoma.

Tonometer Instrument to measure intraocular pressure.

Trabecular meshwork Connective tissue meshwork in the *anterior chamber angle* through which aqueous drains.

Trichiasis Irritation of the cornea by eyelashes.

Vogt-Koyanagi-Harada disease Uveitis, retinal detachment, meningitis, vitiligo, alopecia, poliosis, and hearing loss.

Waardenburg syndrome Telecanthus, heterochromia iridum, white forelock, and congenital deafness.

Wagner vitreoretinal degeneration Dominant hereditary vitreoretinal dystrophy with abnormal vitreous strands, cataract, and retinal detachment. Often associated with generalized connective tissue abnormalities (Stickler syndrome).

Water drinking test Provocative test for glaucoma; the patient drinks one quart of water after fasting, and the intraocular pressure is measured every 15 minutes.

Wegener's granulomatosis Generalized necrotizing vasculitis especially of the respiratory tract and kidney with involvement of the eye (*conjunctivitis, keratitis, uveitis,* retinitis) or orbit (*pseudotumor*) in 50% of cases.

Xanthelasma Yellow plaque on the eyelids due to lipid deposition.

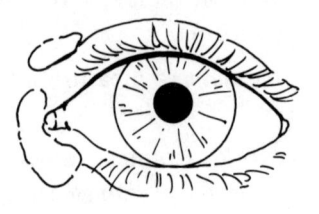

Xanthelasma

Xerophthalmia Dryness of the cornea and conjunctiva due to vitamin A deficiency.

Annotated Bibliography

Duke-Elder S: System of Ophthalmology, 15 vols. St. Louis, Mosby, 1967–1976. *The* authoritative reference in ophthalmology up to the publication date of each volume.

Duane TD (ed): Clinical Ophthalmology. Hagerstown, MD, Harper and Row, 5 volumes with index. Partial yearly revisions. The most-up-to-date comprehensive general reference.

Henkind P, Walsh JB, Berger AW (ed): Physicians Desk Reference for Ophthalmology, Oradell, NJ, Medical Economics Co. (yearly editions). Reference for ophthalmic pharmaceuticals, guide to the evaluation of permanent visual impairment and other useful information.

The Yearbook of Ophthalmology, Oradell, NJ, Medical Economics Co (yearly editions). A selection of articles with editorial comment on current topics of ophthalmologic interest.

Monographs

There are dozens of monographs on every subdivision of ophthalmology. Monographs contain detailed information not available in any single or multivolume general textbook.

Journals

American Journal of Ophthalmology, AMA Archives of Ophthalmology, and *Ophthalmology* are the leading American ophthalmology journals. In these and many other American and international journals you will find the most recent developments in ophthalmology.

Index

Page numbers in **bold face** locate a definition or discussion of the entity; *f* following a page number indicates a figure.

Abbreviations, **16**
Abetalipoproteinemia, 129
Accommodation, 70, 75f, **75-76**
Acetazolamide, 40
Acoustic neuroma, **102**, 161
Actinic keratopathy, 115
Adenoid cystic carcinoma of lacrimal gland, 112
Adenovirus, 45, 48
Adie's pupil, 89 90f, 143
Adnexa oculi, 143
Afferent pupillary defect, 95, 96
Albinism, 5
Alkaptonuria, 116
Allergy, 7, 145
  conjunctivitis due to, 43, 45
Alport syndrome, 129
Alternating hemiplegia, 69
Amaurosis, 143
  fugax, 143
Amaurotic family idiocy, 132
Amblyopia, **143**, 157
  ex anopsia, 81, 162
Amblyoscope, 84
Ametropia, 74
Amiodarone, 116
Amphotericin B, 49
Amyloid degeneration of cornea, 115

Anesthetic, topical, 17, 23, 25, 27, **38**
Angioid streaks, 130, 132, **143**
Anisocoria, 90f, **143**
Anterior chamber, **55**, 162
  abnormalities of, 6f
  function of, 4f
Anterior chamber angle, 138, 144, 167
Anterior chamber cleavage syndrome, **144**
Anterior segment, **144**
  mesenchymal dysgenesis of, **144**
Antibiotics
  eyedrops, 35-37
  systemic, **37**
Antiviral eyedrops, **40**
Aphakia, **144**, 154
Aphakic bullous keratopathy, 116, **144**, 146
Applanation tonometer, 118f, **119**
Aqueous flare and cells, 51
Arcus senilis, **144**, 152f
Argyll Robertson pupil, 89, 100, 132, **144**
Arrhythmias, 39
Arteries
  carotid, 66, 143, 163
  posterior inferior cerebellar, 68-69

173

Arteries (continued)
  retinal, 3, 33, 65f, **65–66**
  vertebral basilar, **67, 68,** 69
Arteriosclerosis, 61, 68
Arteriovenous compression, 60, 61
Asteroid hyalosis, 145
Astigmatism, 70, 73f, **73–74,** 74f, 118
Ataxia telangiectasia, 129
Atherosclerosis, 143, 146
Atopic dermatitis, 129
Atropine, 39
AV nicking, 60
Axenfield syndrome, 144
Axial hyperopia, 75
Axial length of eye, 74–75
Axial myopia, 75

Bacitracin, 36
Band keratopathy, 116
Basal cell carcinoma, **104,** 105f, 133
Bassen-Kornzweig syndrome, 129
Behçet syndrome, 53, **145**
Bell's phenomenon, 145
Benedikt syndrome, 68
Benoxinate, 38
Beri-beri, 129
Berlin's edema, **145**
Best's vitelliform degeneration, 134
Biber corneal dystrophy, 115

Bielschowsky sign, 83
Binocular vision, 84
Bitot's spot, 132, **145**
Blepharitis, **7,** 28f, **32,** 48, 148
Blepharochalasis, 103, **145**
Blepharophimosis, **145**
Blepharoptosis, **103,** 104f, **145,** 157
Blepharospasm, **145**
Blind spot, 56, **145**
Blindness, 62, 65, 143, 163
  legal, 3
  night, **7,** 129, 132, 147, 163
  river, 131
  total, 9
Bloch-Sulzberger syndrome, 130
Blowout fracture of orbit, 5, **21–22**
Bourneville disease, **161**
Bowman's membrane, 53, 117f
Brain stem syndromes, **68–69,** 100
Brain tumors, **99–102**
  symptoms and signs of, **100–102**
Brittle bones, **131**
Brown syndrome, **145–146**
Bulbar, defined, **146**
Bullous keratopathy, **146**
Buphthalmos, **146**
Busacca nodules, 51

Caldwell-Luc antrotomy, 114
Canal of Schlemm, 55, **146**

Index

Canthus, 20f, **146**
Capillary hemangioma, 104
Capsulotomy, 87
Carcinoma
   adenoid cystic, of lacrimal
      gland, 112
   basal cell, of eyelids, **104**,
      105f, **133**
   squamous cell, of eyelids,
      104, 105f, **133**
Carotid arteriography, 66
Carotid artery, occlusion of,
   66–67
Carotid bruit, 66
Carotid-cavernous fistula, 5,
   146
Carotid endarterectomy, 66
Cataract, 3, 7, 14, 59, 77,
   85–88, **129–132**, 140,
   153, 154
   congenital, **87**
   cortical, 85, 86f
   extraction of
      extracapsular, **85**, 86f
      intracapsular, **85**, 148
   in galactosemia, 130
   mature, 86f
   nuclear, 85, 86f
   posterior subcapsular, 85
   sunflower, 132
   traumatic, 87
Cavernous hemangioma, 111
Cavernous sinus thrombosis, 5,
   30, **31**
Cellulitis, orbital, 5, **29–30**, 37
Central retinal artery occlusion,
   65, 65f
Central retinal vein occlusion,
   64, 64f
Central serous
   chorioretinopathy, 7,
   146–47
Ceramide trihexoside, 130
Cerebellar ataxia, 129
Cerebellar medulloblastoma, 101
Cerebellopontine angle tumor,
   161
Chalazion, **32**
Chalcosis, 26
Chamber. *See* Anterior
   chamber; Posterior
   chamber
Charcot's traid, 98
Chemosis, 131, 146, **147**
Chlamydia, 33, 46, **147**
Chloroquine, 116
Chorioretinitis, **53**, 132
   presumed histoplasmic,
      123–124, 124f
Choroid
   abnormalities of, 6f
   function of, 4f
   melanoma of, 77, **108**
   neovascularization of, 121
Choroidal detachment, **147**
Choroideremia, **147**, 153
Choroiditis, 6f, **51**
Chronic progressive
   ophthalmoplegia, 158
Ciliary body
   abnormalities of, 6f
   function of, 4f
Ciliary injection, 28, 43, 44f,
   51, 58

Index

Circinate retinopathy, 147
Circumpapillary, 148
Clindamycin, 123
Cogan corneal dystrophy, 115
Cogan syndrome, 129
Collagen disease, 116
Collyrium, 38
Coloboma, 131, 147, 154f
Congenital cataract, 87
Congenital glaucoma, 58
Compresses, 35
Computed tomography, 109, 135, 136f
Conjunctiva
   bulbar, 43, 44f
   foreign bodies of, 5, 24–25, 25f
   palpebral, 20f, 43
   shrinkage of, 131
   telangiectasia of, 129
Conjunctivitis, 3, 5, 19–20, 43–47, 44f, 131, 155, 163, 167
   acute, 18
   acute catarrhal, 43
   chlamydial, 33, 46, 147
   chronic, 46
   follicular, 43, 44f
   gonorrheal, 33, 46
   inclusion, 46, 147
   of newborn, 33
   membranous, 46–47
   papillary, 43, 44f
   Parinaud's 45
   swimming pool, 45, 46
   vernal, 45f, 45–46, 129

Conjunctivodacryocystorhinostomy, 107
Contact lenses, 43, 77, 140, 155
   three mirror, 119
Convergence, 70, 82
Corectopia, 147, 154f
Cornea, 20f, 115–119, 140
   abnormalities of, 6f, 48f, 152f
   abrasion of, 5, 48f
   anesthesia of, 69
   beaded nerves of, 116
   chemical burns of, 27
   crystals in, 116, 129
   degeneration of, 115,
   disease of, 19, 23–24, 48f
   dysgenesis of, 115
   dystrophy of, 58, 115, 152f, 155
   vortex, 116, 130
   effect of damage to, 117f
   endothelium of, 150, 151
   epithelium of, 17
   erosion of, 48
   foreign bodies in, 5, 25, 28f, 119
   function of, 4f
   guttata, 115
   haze, 116
   injury to, 19, 23–24
   Kayser-Fleischer rings of, 116, 133, 155
   laceration of, 24f
   layers of, 117f
   limbus of, 20f, 51, 144, 148
   lipid infiltration of, 144
   melting of, 116

plana, 115
stroma, 117f
surgery of, 116–118
in systemic disease, 116
transplantation of, 116–117, 155
ulcers of, 26, 27, 47–49, 48f, 131
fungal, 49
uric acid crystals in, 116
Cotton wool spots, 60, 130, 131
Cranial arteritis, 96–97
Cranial nerve palsy, 83, 103
Cranial nerves, 5
third, 83, 90, 103, 165
fourth, 83, 165
fifth, 7, 131
sixth, 83, 131, 165
seventh, 69, 131
twelfth, 69
Craniopharyngioma, 102
Crohn's disease, 129
Cromolyn, 46
Crouzon syndrome, 148
Crystalline degeneration of cornea, 115
CT scan, 109, 135, 136f
Cultures, 35
Cyclitis, 125
Cyclopentolate, 39
Cycloplegics, 39, 71
Cylinder, 73, 148
Cystinosis, 116, 129
Cystoid macular edema, 87, 148
Cytomegalovirus inclusion disease, 129

Dacryocystitis, 31, 105
Dacrycystorhinostomy, 107
Deafness, 129, 131, 158, 163, 167
Decongestants, 38
Degenerations of cornea, 115
Demodex folliculorum, 7, 148
Depth perception, 84
Dermatomyositis, 130
Dermoid cyst, 111
Descemetocele, 48f
Descemet's membrane, 117f
Detachment
of retina. *See* Retinal detachment
of vitreous, 127
Diabetic retinopathy, 60, 62–63, 62f, 63f,134,164
proliferative, 63, 63f, 126–128, 138
Diagnosis, 17
Diagnostic studies of eye, 134–137
Diopters, 70, 76
prism, 79
Dipivefrin, 40, 148
Diplopia, 5, 129, 157
monocular, 5
Disciform macular degeneration, 120, 121f, 155
Discission, 87
Dislocated lens, 130, 148, 154
Disseminated hamartomas, 160
Distichiasis, 148
Divergence, 70
Double vision, 5

Drusen, 120, 121f, 148, 149f
Duane syndrome, 149
Dyslexia, 141, 149
Dysmetric eye movements, 69
Dystrophy, corneal, 58, 115, 152f, 155

Ectodermal dysplasia, 132
Ectropion, 103, 149f, 149–150
Edrophonium, 157
Ehlers-Danlos syndrome, 130, 143
Eightball hemorrhage, 21
Electro-oculogram 134, 135f
Electroretinogram, 7, 134, 135f
Embryotoxon, 131, 150
Emmetrope, 150
Emmetropia, 72
Endarterectomy, carotid, 66
Endophthalmitis, 26, 125, 150
Endothelium, 117f, 150, 151
Enophthalmos, 114, 128, 149, 150
Entropion, 46, 103, 150, 150f
Enucleation, 151
Epicanthus, 145, 151
Epikeratophakia, 117
Epiphora, 151. *See also* Tearing
Episcleritis, 28f, 29, 50, 129, 131
Esotropia, 16, 78, 79, 80f, 80–81
  accommodative, 81
  alternating, 80
  constant, 81

Essential hypertension, 60
Essential iris atrophy, 151, 154f
Evisceration, 151
Exenteration, 30, 151
Exophthalmometry, 109f
Exophthalmos, 108–109, 110f, 146, 150
Exotropia, 16, 78, 79, 80f, 81–82
External disease, 43–50
Extraocular muscle palsy, 5, 78, 82–84, 89
Exudates, cotton-wool, 130, 131
Eye and eyeball
  abnormalities of, 6f
  compresses for, 35
  contusion of, 21, 28f
  crusted, 7
  cultures, 35
  diagnosis of emergencies, 17
  diagnostic studies of, 134–137
  dry, 5, 155
  emergencies, 17–33
  examination of, 3–16
  external
    examinations, 12–13
    structures, 20f
  function of, 4f
  history taking, 3, 17
  inflammation of, 5, 26, 32, 150, 160
  injury to 14, 19
    penetrating, 22–23
  landmarks of, 20f
  lazy. *See* Strabismus
  misunderstandings about, 140–141

ointments, 34, 35–37
painful, 5, 140
patches, 34–35
pharmacology, 34–40
phthisical, 162
pink. *see* Conjunctivitis
"quiet," 33
red, 3, 18–19
red rimmed, 7
reduced, 70
rupture of, 21, 22
schematic, 70
spots before, 7
symptoms involving, 3–8
systemic disease and, 129–133
trauma to, 21
treatment of emergencies, 17
vascular disease and, 59, 60
Eyedrops, 34,
administration of, 36f
anesthetic, 38
antibiotic, 35–36
antiviral, 40
cycloplegic, 39
mydriatic, 39
steroid, 37
Eyeglasses, 77
Eyelids, 103–104
diseases of, 103
eversion of, 130
heliotrope discoloration of, 130
involuntary closure of, 145
laceration of, 23
retraction of, 103
surgery, 103
tumors of, 104, 105f, 133

twitching, 8
Eyewash, 38, 140

Fabry's disease, 116, 130
Field. *See* Visual field
Filtering operation, 56
Fissure
sphenoidal, 159, 165
superior orbital, 165
"Flashburn," 26–27
Fluorescein, 151
angiography, 119, 134, 151
stain, 17
strip, 23, 151
Follicles, 43, 44f, 46
Foreign body, 3, 24
conjunctival, 5, 24–25, 25f
corneal, 5, 25, 28f, 119
intraocular, 22, 26, 128
sensation, 5
spud, 25f
Foster-Kennedy syndrome, 99–100
pseudo–, 96
Foville syndrome, 68
Fracture
long bone, 130
orbital, 21–22, 114
blowout, 5, 21–22
tripod, 21
Francheschetti syndrome, 131
Fuchs corneal dystrophy, 115, 116, 146, 151, 152f
Fundus, 152
Furrow degeneration of cornea, 115
Fusion, 84

180 Index

Galactosemia, 130
Gentamicin, 35
Gerstmann syndrome, 100
Glands
  meibomian, 32, 148
  tarsal, 32
Glaucoma, 3, 55–59, 151, 167
  acute congestive, 3, 19, 24f,
    29, 43, 58, 89, 90f, 141,
    144
  chronic simple, 11, 55–56
  congenital, 58
  cupping of optic disc in, 56f
  diagnosis of, 55
  low tension, 59
  medications for, 39–40
  narrow-angle, 7, 14, 29,
    57–58, 144, 154
  open-angle, 29, 55–56, 138
  screening tests for, 55
  secondary, 53, 54, 58, 63, 87,
    108, 138, 163
  visual field loss in, 57f
Glioblastoma multiforme,
    100–101
Glioma, optic nerve, 112
Globe, 152. *See also* Eye and
  eyeball
  contusion of, 21, 89
  rupture of, 21, 22
Goldenhar syndrome, 152
Goldman-Favre disease, 152–53
Gonorrheal ophthalmia, 33, 46
Gonioscopic lens, 138, 153
Gonioscopy, 153
Goniotomy, 58
Gout, 116

Gramicidin, 36
Granular degeneration of
  cornea, 115
Graves' disease, 5, 110f
Groenouw corneal dystrophy,
  115
Grönblad-Strandberg
  syndrome, 132
Gyrate atrophy, 153

Haloes, 7
Hamartoma, 153, 160
Hard exudates, 60, 63
Headache, 146
  cluster, 153
  tension, 5
  vascular, 5
Hemangioma, 133
  cavernous, 111
Hemianopsia, homonymous,
  66, 67, 101f
Hemiplegia, 68, 69
Hemorrhage
  blot, 60, 63
  flame-shaped, 60
  retinal, 130, 131
  subconjunctival, 3, 18, 20–21
  vitreous, 3, 7, 63, 128, 138
Hepatolenticular degeneration,
  133
Herpes simplex keratitis, 48–49
Herpes zoster, 49, 50f
Heterochromia of iris, 153, 167
Heterophoria, 79

Index

Heterotropia, 79
Hirschberg test, 78
Histoplasmic chorioretinitis, 123–24, 124f
Histoplasmosis, 120, 124f, 138
Hollenhorst plaques, 67
Homocystinuria, 130, 148
Homonymous hemianopsia, 66, 67, 101f
Hordeolum, 32
Horner syndrome, 89, 90f, 91–93, 92f, 103, 143, 153, 162
Horton syndrome, 5, 93, 153
Hruby lens, 119
Hypercalcemia, 116
Hyperostosis, 102
Hyperlipoproteinemia, 130
Hyperopia, 70, 72, 73f, 74f, 140, 165
   axial, 75
Hypertelorism, 148, 153, 166
Hypertropia, 78, 80f, 82
Hyphema, 21
Hypoparathyroidism, 130
Hypopion, 28, 47, 48f, 53, 145
Hypotony, 97, 147, 153
Hypotropia, 78, 82

Idoxuridine, 40
Inclusion conjunctivitis, 46, 147
Incontinenta pigmenti, 130
Indirect ophthalmoscopy, 127, 158

Internuclear opthalmoplegia, 98
Interstitial keratitis, 116, 129, 131, 132, 152f, 153
Intracranial calcification, 122
Intraocular foreign body, 22, 26, 128
Intraocular lens, 14, 87–88, 88f
Intraocular pressure, 16, 17, 59
   elevated, 55
   low. *See* Hypotony
   measurement of, 59, 167
Iridectomy, 29, 58, 154, 154f
Iridocyclitis, 51, 53, 59, 116
Iridodialysis, 154, 154f
Iridodonesis, 154
Iridotomy, 29, 154f, 154–55
   laser, 58
Iris, 20f, 140
   abnormalities of, 6f, 154f
   bombé, 52f, 53
   function of, 4f
   heterochromia of, 153, 167
   nodules in, 51
   pupillary margin of, 51
Iritis, 19, 28–29, 51, 52f, 53, 89, 90f, 153. *See also* Uveitis
   acute, 24f
   anterior, 51
Ischemia optic neuropathy
   anterior, 95–96
   posterior, 96

Juvenile retinoschisis, 155

Kayser-Fleischer ring, 116, 133, 155
Kearns-Sayre syndrome, 158, 163
Keratinoid degeneration of cornea, 115
Keratitis, 3, 5, 130, 155, 167
  contact lens, 27, 48
  dendritic, 48–49
  fungal, 37, 49
  herpetic, 24f, 48–49, 129
  interstitial, 116, 129, 131, 132, 152f, 153
  superficial punctate, 27, 47–48, 48f
  ultraviolet, 26–27
Keratoconjunctivitis, 44
  epidemic, 45
  sicca, 48, 155, 164
Keratoconus, 117, 129, 131, 155
Keratoglobus, 115
Keratomalacia, 132
Keratopathy
  actinic, 115
  aphakic bullous, 116, 144, 146
  band, 53, 132
  bullous, 145
  Labrador, 115
Keratoplasty
  lamellar, 117
  penetrating, 116–17
  refractive, 117–18
Keratoprosthesis, 155
Keratotomy, radial, 117
Koeppe nodules, 51

Kronlein orbitotomy, 114
Kuhnt-Junius disease, 155

Labrador keratopathy, 115
Laceration
  of cornea, 24f
  of eyelid, 23
  of tear duct, 23
Lacrimal canaliculi, 105
Lacrimal duct, 106
Lacrimal gland
  adenoid cystic carcinoma of, 112
  mixed tumor of, 112
Lacrimal intubation, 106–107
Lacrimal puncta, 105, 120f
Lacrimal system, 105–107, 106f
  diseases of, 103
  obstruction of, 105
  surgery on, 103
Lagophthalmos, 103, 155
Lamellar, definition of, 155
Lamellar keratoplasty, 117
Laser, 19, 138–139
  argon, 138
  capsulotomy, 87
  CO_2, 139
  iridotomy, 119, 154f
  krypton, 138
  neodynium-YAG, 139
  photocoagulation, 122
  trabeculoplasty, 119
  YAG, 139
Lateral medullary syndrome, 68–69

Index

Lateral rectus palsy, 83
Lattice degeneration
  of cornea, 155
  of retina, 156
Laurence-Moon-Biedl
  syndrome, 130
Lazy eye. *See* Strabismus
Leber's hereditary optic
  atrophy, 156
Legal blindness
  benefits for legally blind, 3
  definition of, 3
Lens
  abnormalities, 6. *See also*
    Cataract
  capsule, 85, 87
  concave, 70
  contact. *See* Contact lenses
  convex, 70, 72
  cortex, 85, 86f
  cylindrical, 73, 148
  dislocated, 130, 148, 154
  function of, 4f
  Hruby, 119
  implant, 87–88, 88f
  minus, 70, 165
  nucleus, 85, 86f
  plus, 72, 165
  spherical, 165
  toric, 73, 75
Lenticonus, anterior, 129
Leprosy, 53, 116, 131
Leukemia, 131
Leukocoria, 156
Leukoma, 152f, 156
Light
  convergence, 70
  divergence, 70
  flashes, 7, 127
  perception of, 9
  projection of, 9
  rays, 70
  ultraviolet, 77, 162
Limbus, corneal, 51, 20f, 144, 148
  pigmentation of, 116
Lipemia retinalis, 130
Lipid degeneration of cornea, 115
Locked-in syndrome, 67
Louis-Bar syndrome, 129
Lupus erythematosus, 131
Lymphogranuloma venereum, 46, 147
Lymphoma of orbit, 113

Macular degeneration
  of cornea, 115
  of retina, 3, 16, 77, 120–122, 134, 138
    age-related, 120–122
    disciform, 120–122, 121f
    dry, 120
    exudative, 120–122
    geographic, 120
    involutional, 120
    nonexudative, 120
    senile, 120–122
    wet, 120–122
Macular drusen, 120, 121f, 148, 149f

Magnetic resonance imaging, 135–136
Mandibulofacial dysostosis, 131
Manzotti reaction, 131
Marcus Gunn phenomenon, 156
Marcus Gunn pupil, 95
Marfan syndrome, 148
Medullated nerve fibers, 157
Meesman corneal dystrophy, 115
Megalocornea, 58, 115, 131
Melanosis oculi, 156
Meniere's disease, 91
Meningioma, 111–112
   intraorbital, 112
   sphenoidal ridge, 102, 111
   tuberculum sellae, 95, 102, 111
Mesenchymal dysgenesis of anterior segment, 144
Metamorphopsia, 7, 146
Methazolamide, 40
Methycellulose, 38
Microaneurysms, 62–63
Microcornea, 115
Microphthalmos, 156
Migraine, 5, 7, 93, 143
Miosis, 89, 90f
Mixed tumor of lacrimal gland, 112
Moebius syndrome, 131
Mohs fresh-tissue surgery, 104, 156
Mooren's ulcer of cornea, 115
Mucocele, 111
Mucopolysaccharidosis, 58, 116, 156

Mucor, 30
Mucormycosis, 5, 30
Multiple myeloma, 131
Multiple sclerosis, 91, 95, 98
Myasthenia gravis, 157
Mydriasis, 89–90, 90f, 158
Mydriatics, 39
Myelinated nerve fibers, 157, 157f
Myokymia, 8
Myopia, 70, 72, 73f, 74f, 118, 140, 157, 165
   axial, 75
Myotonic dystrophy, 157

Nasal step, 56f
Nasolacrimal duct, 106f
Near point of convergence, 82
Neomycin, 36
Neovascularization
   of iris, 138
   of peripheral retina, 163
   subretinal, 121, 124, 138
Nerve palsy, 83, 103. *See also* Cranial nerves
Neuritis
   optic, 94, 131
   retrobulbar, 94
Neuroblastoma, adrenal, 114
Neurofibromatosis, 161
Neurons, 92–93
Neuro-ophthalmology, 89–102
Neuropathy, 131
   ischemic optic, 95–96

Index   185

anterior, 95–96
posterior, 96
trigeminal, 5
Night blindness, 7, 129, 132,
    147, 163
Nonrhegmatogenous retinal
    detachment, 126–27
Nuclei, cranial nerve, 68, 69
Nystagmus, 69, 90–91, 129
    dissociated, 91
    end position, 91
    jerk, 91
    latent, 91
    optokinetic, 159
    pendular, 91
    railroad, 91
    vestibular, 91

Occlusion
    branch vein, 11, 63, 64–65
    carotid, 66, 143, 163
    central retinal arery, 3, 33,
        65f, 65–66
    central retinal vein, 3, 33, 59,
        64–65, 131, 132, 134,
        138, 164
    middle cerebral artery, 66
    vertebral-basilar, 67
Ocular adnexa, 17
Ocular media, 5, 14
Ocular trauma, 128
Ocular tumors, 107–108
Ocularist, 157
Oculist, 158

Oculo-auriculo-vertebral
    dysplasia, 152
Oculomotor apraxia, 129
Oculoplastic surgery, 103, 139
Oculus, 158
Onchocerciasis, 131
Ophthalmia
    gonorrheal, 46
    neonatorum, 32–33
    sympathetic, 53, 165
Ophthalmic herpes zoster, 49,
    50
Ophthalmic plastic surgery,
    103, 139
Ophthalmo-, definition of, 158
Ophthalmodynamometer, 66
Ophthalmologist, 158
Ophthalmopathy, thyroid, 110,
    110f, 114
Ophthalmoplegia, 158, 163
    external, 83, 158
    internal, 89, 158
    internuclear, 98
    "plus," 158
    progressive external, 158
    total, 83, 89, 158
Ophthalmoscopy, 13–16
    direct, 14, 159
    examination by, 14f
    indirect, 127, 158–159
Optic abnormalities, 66f
Optic atrophy, 94f, 130, 159
    Leber's, 156
Optic chiasm, 99f
Optic disc, 55, 56f
Optic nerve, 4f, 6f
    glioma, 112

Optic neuritis or neuropathy,
11, 94–95, 98
  anterior ischemic, 95–96
  posterior ischemic, 96
  retrobulbar, 96
Optician, 159
Optics, 70
Optokinetic drum, 91, 159
Optokinetic nystagmus, 91
Optometrist, 159
Orbit
  computed tomography of,
  135
  decompression of, 114
  diseases of, 108–111
  fractures of, 21–22, 114
    blowout, 5, 21–22
    tripod, 21
  lymphoma of, 113
  pseudotumors of, 5,
  110–111, 167
  reconstruction of, 114
  surgery of, 114
  tumors of, 5, 97, 111–14
  secondary, 113
Orbital apex syndrome, 159
Orbital cellulitis, 29–30, 30f
Orbitotomy, 114
Orthoptics, 84
Orthoptist, 84
Osteogenesis imperfecta, 131
Osteopath, 160

Pachometer, 119
Paget's disease, 143

Palsy. *See* Nerve palsy
Pannus, 46, 152f
Panophthalmitis, 160
Panretinal photocoagulation,
138
Papillae, cobblestone, 45
Papillary, definition of, 160
Papilledema, 97, 97f, 98f, 143
Papillitis, 97
Parinaud (midbrain) syndrome,
100
Parinaud oculoglandular
  syndrome, 44–45
Pellucid marginal degeneration
  of cornea, 115
Pemphigoid, 131
Penicillin, 46
Perimeter, 160
Peripapillary, definition of, 160
Peters anomaly, 144
Phacomatoses, 160–61
Pharmacology of eye, 34–40
Pharyngoconjunctival fever, 45
Phenylephrine hydrochloride,
39
Phoria, 79
Phoropter, 71
Photocoagulation, laser, 138
Photophobia, 5
Photopsia, 7
Phthisis bulbi, 161
Pilocarpine, 40, 90f
Pimaricin, 49
Pinguecula, 161, 161f
Pinhole disc, 9, 10f
Pink eye. *See* Conjunctivitis
Pituitary adenoma, 101–102
Polyarteritis nodosa, 132

Index

Polycythemia, 132
Polymyxin, 36
Polyvinyl alcohol, 38
Posterior chamber, 162
Posterior pole, 162
Presbyopia, 75f, **76**
Prisms, 77
    in diagnosis of strabismus, 79
Prism diopters, 79
Proliferative diabetic
    retinopathy, **63**, 126, 127, 128, 138
Proparacaine, 38
Proptosis, **5**, 31, 108, 131, 150
Pseudo–Foster-Kennedy syndrome, **96**
Pseudomembranes, 47
Pseudopapilledema, 72
Pseudoptosis, 162
Pseudostrabismus, 162
Pseudotumor, orbital, **5**, 110–111, 167
Pseudoxanthoma elasticum, 132, 143
Psittacosis, 46
Pterygium, 77, 117, 152f, **162**
Ptosis, **103**, 130, 156
    eyebrow, 103
Pupil
    Adie's, 89, 90f, **143**
    afferent defect of, **95**
    anisocoria, 90f, **143**
    Argyll Robertson, 89, 100, 132, **144**
    consensual reaction of, 89
    constriction of, **89**
    dilation of, 13–14
    Horner, 90f, **93**

Marcus Gunn, 95
miosis, **89**, 90f
mydriasis, **89–90**, 90f, 158
near reaction, 86
Purtscher's retinopathy, 130
Pyrimethamine, 123

Racemose hemangioma of retina, 133
Radial keratotomy, 117
Radiation, 108, 113
Raeder syndrome, 93, 162
Red eye, **3**, 19
Reduced eye, 164
Refraction, 70–71
    error of, 70, 74–75
    manifest, 71
Refsum syndrome, 163
Reiger syndrome, 144
Reis-Buckler corneal dystrophy, 115
Reiter syndrome, 163
Retina, **120–127**
    abnormalities of, 6f
    arteriolar pulsation of, 16, 66
    artery occlusion in, **3**, 33, **65–66**, 65f
    Berlin's edema of, **145**
    branch vein occlusion in, 11, 63, **64–65**
    breaks in, **125**
    dysplasia of, 130
    function of, 4f
    hemorrhage, 130, 131
    holes in, 7

Retina (continued)
  irreversible vascular changes
    in, 60
  landmarks of, 15f
  photocoagulation of, 138
  mulberry tumors of, 161
  reversible vascular changes
    in, 60
  tears in, 125, 127
  vascular disease of, 60–63
  vasculitis of, 132
  vein occlusion in, 3, 33, 59,
    64–65, 64f, 131, 132,
    134, 138, 164
  venous pulsation of, 15–16
Retinal detachment, 3, 7, 11,
    87, 125–127, 126f, 128,
    167
  exudative, 127
  nonrhegmatogenous,
    126–127
  rhegmatogenous, 125–126
  traction, 63, 126–127, 128,
    138, 163
Retinal pigment epithelium,
    120, 134
Retinitis, 129
  of prematurity, 163
Retinitis pigmentosa, 7, 130,
    131, 153, 156, 163
Retinoblastoma, 79, 107–108, 124
Retinochoroiditis, 122, 123f
Retinopathy
  background, 62
  circinate, 147
  diabetic. See Diabetic
    retinopathy
  grading of, 61
  hypertensive, 60, 61f, 62f
  pigmentary, 129
  proliferative, 63, 63f, 132
  Purtscher's, 130
Retinoschisis, 153, 163
  juvenile, 155
Retinoscopy, 70
Retrobulbar neuritis, 94
Retrolental fibroplasia, 126, 163
Rhabdomyosarcoma, 113
Rhegmatogenous retinal
    detachment, 125–126
River blindness, 131
Rollet syndrome, 159
Roth spots, 131, 163–164, 164f
Rothmund Thompson
    syndrome, 132
Rubeosis iridis, 59, 63, 64, 138,
    164

Salzman nodular degeneration
    of cornea, 115
Sarcoidosis, 53
Schematic eye, 164
Schiøtz tonometry, 17, 18f, 59
Schirmer test, 164
Schnyder corneal dystrophy,
    115
Sclera
  abnormalities of, 6f
  blue, 130, 131
  diseases of, 49–50
  function of, 4f
  pigmentation of, 116

Index

Scleritis, 29, 131
  deep, 49–50
  episcleritis, 50
  nodular, 49–50
Sclerocornea, 115
Scleroderma, 132
Scleromalacia perforans, 50
Scotoma, 164
  Bjerrum, 56, 57f
  central, 129
  scintillating, 93
  Seidel, 56
Seborrhea, 7
Senile macular degeneration, 120–122
Sickle cell disease, 132, 143
Siderosis, 26
Silicone intubation, 106–107
Sinusitis, 5
Sjögren syndrome, 132, 155, 164
Slit lamp, 118–119, 118f
Snellen eye chart, 8–9, 11
Speed reading, 165
Sphenoidal fissure syndrome 159, 165
Sphere, 165
  minus, 165
  plus, 165
Spheroidal degeneration of cornea, 115
Squamous carcinoma of the eyelid, 104, 105f, 133
Squint, *See* Strabismus
Staphylococcus infection, 7, 43
Staphyloma, 165
Stargardt disease, 165

Stereopsis, 84
Steroid eye medications, 37
Stevens-Johnson disease, 47
Stickler syndrome, 167
Still's disease, 53, 132
Strabismus, 3, 78–84, 91, 130, 157
  comitant, 78
  diagnosis of, 78
  incomitant, 78, 82–84
  treatment of, 84
Stroke, 66, 69
Sturge-Weber syndrome, 161
Stye, 32
Subclavian steal syndrome, 67
Subconjunctival hemorrhage, 3, 18, 20–21
Subretinal neovascularization, 121, 124, 138
Sulfacetamide, 35
Sulfadiazine, 123
Sulfisoxazole, 32
Superficial punctate keratitis, 47–48, 48f
Superior oblique palsy, 83
Superior oblique tendon sheath syndrome, 145–146
Suppression, 78, 80
Symblepharon, 103, 131, 165
Sympathetic ophthalmia, 165
Synchysis scintilans, 165–166
Synechia
  anterior, 52f, 53
  posterior, 51, 52f
Syneresis of vitreous, 127
Synkinesis, 76
Syphilis, 53, 116, 132, 148

Talosa-Hunt syndrome, 166
Tangent screen, 166, 166f
Tarsal glands, 32
Tarsorrhaphy, 166
Tarsus, 166
Tay Sachs disease, 132
Tearing, 7, 151
  bilateral, 151
  chronic, 7
  unilateral, 7, 151
Tears
  artificial, 38
  overproduction of, 107
  reduced secretion of, 5, 155
Telecanthus, 145, 153, 166, 167
Temporal arteritis, 96–97
Terrien's marginal
  degeneration of cornea,
  115
Tests
  cover-uncover, 79
  enzyme-linked
    immunosorbent assay
    (ELISA), 124
  Hirschberg, 78
Tetracaine, 38
Tetracycline, 32
Tetrahydrozoline, 38
Thygeson-superficial punctate
  keratitis, 48
Thyroid disease, 108, 110
  exophthalmos in, 108
  eyelid retraction in, 110
  ophthalmopathy of, 110, 114
Timolol, 39–40
Tobramycin, 32
Tonography, 167

Tonometer, 167
  applanation, 118f, 119
  Schiøtz, 17, 18f, 59
Toxemia of pregnancy, 60
Toxocara canis, 124–125
Toxocariasis, 120, 124–125
Toxoplasmosis, 120, 122–123
Trabecular meshwork, 55, 57,
  146, 167
Trabeculoplasty, laser, 56, 138
Trachoma, 46, 147
Transient ischemic attacks, 66
Trantas' dots, 45
Treacher-Collins syndrome,
  131
Trial case, 70
Trial frame, 70
Trichiasis, 46, 103, 150, 167
Trifluorothymidine, 40
Trigeminal neuropathy, 5
Tropia, 79
Tropicamide, 39, 90f
Tuberculosis, 53
Tuberous sclerosis, 161
Tumors
  basal cell, of eyelid, 104,
    105f, 133
  brain, 99–102
  brain stem, 100
  cavernous hemangioma, 111
  choroidal melanoma, 77, 108
  eyelid, 104, 105f, 133
  frontal lobe, 99–100
  hamartomatous, 153, 160
  intraocular, 59, 107–108,
    113, 134
  metastatic, 113–114

Index

mixed, of lacrimal gland, 112
occipital lobe, 100
ocular, 107–108
orbital, 5, 97, 111–114
parietal lobe, 100
retinoblastoma, 79, 107–108, 124
squamous cell, of eyelid, 104, 105f, 133
temporal lobe, 100

Ultrasonogram, 136f, 137f
Ultrasound, 109, 136–137
Ultraviolet light, 77, 162
 keratitis, 26–27
Uveitis, 3, 43, 51–54, 52f, 129–131, 145, 163, 167
 anterior nongranulomatous, 51
 granulomatous, 53
 posterior, 53
 treatment of, 54

Van der Hoeve syndrome, 131
Vertebral-basilar artery occlusion, 67
Vidarabine, 40
Virus, herpes simplex, 48–49
Vision
 binocular, 84
 central, 8–10, 17
 double, 5
 finger count, 9
 hand motion, 9
 light perception, 9
 light projection, 9
 no light perception, 9
 peripheral, 10, 17
 requirements for driving, 3
 stereoscopic, 84
Visual acuity, 8–12
Visual evoked potential, 135, 135f
Visual field, 10
 central, 12f
 confrontation, 10, 11f
 defects of, 11–12
  altitudinal, 11, 95
  glaucomatous, 55, 57f
  hemianopsia, 66, 67
  homonymous, 101f
  monocular, 12f
  quadrantic, 12f
  segmental, 12f
 peripheral, 10, 12f
Visual loss
 with pain, 3
 painless, 3, 33
 sudden, 3, 63, 64, 65
Vitamin A deficiency, 132, 145, 168
Vitamin B deficiency, 129
Vitrectomy, 26, 63, 127–28, 128f
Vitreoretinal degeneration, 152
 Wagner, 167
Vitreous, 127–28
 abnormalities of, 6f

Vitreous (*continued*)
  detachment, 127
  floaters, 7, 14, 16
  function of, 4f
  hemorrhage, 3, 7, 63, 128, 138
  syneresis, 127
Vogt-Koyanhagi-Harada disease, 167
Von Hippel-Landau disease, 161
Von Recklinghausen disease, 161
Vortex corneal dystrophy, 116, 130

Wallenberg syndrome, 68–69, 91
Water drinking test, 167
Water's view, 22
Weber syndrome, 68
Wegener's granulomatosis, 167
Wernicke's encephalopathy, 129
Wilson's disease, 116, 133, 155
Wyburn-Mason syndrome, 133

Xanthelasma, 130, 168
Xeroderma pigmentosum, 133
Xerophthalmia, 132, 168

Waardenburg syndrome, 167
Wagner vitreoretinal degeneration, 167
Waldenstrom's macroglobulinemia, 132

Zinc sulfate, 38
Zonules
  abnormalities of, 6f
  function of, 4f